NEUROLOGY FOR
THE HOSPITALIST

NEUROLOGY FOR THE HOSPITALIST

A Practical Approach

David Likosky, MD, SFHM
EvergreenHealth Medical Center

S. Andrew Josephson, MD
University of California San Francisco

Michael J. Pistoria, DO, FACP, SFHM
Lehigh Valley Health Network

W. David Freeman, MD
Mayo Clinic

OXFORD
UNIVERSITY PRESS

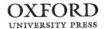

OXFORD

UNIVERSITY PRESS

Oxford University Press is a department of the University of Oxford.
It furthers the University's objective of excellence in research, scholarship,
and education by publishing worldwide.

Oxford   New York
Auckland   Cape Town   Dar es Salaam   Hong Kong   Karachi
Kuala Lumpur   Madrid   Melbourne   Mexico City   Nairobi
New Delhi   Shanghai   Taipei   Toronto

With offices in
Argentina   Austria   Brazil   Chile   Czech Republic   France   Greece
Guatemala   Hungary   Italy   Japan   Poland   Portugal   Singapore
South Korea   Switzerland   Thailand   Turkey   Ukraine   Vietnam

Oxford is a registered trademark of Oxford University Press
in the UK and certain other countries.

Published in the United States of America by
Oxford University Press
198 Madison Avenue, New York, NY 10016

Library of Congress Cataloging-in-Publication Data
Likosky, David J., author.
Neurology for the Hospitalist : A Practical Approach / David Likosky, S. Andrew Josephson, Michael
Joseph Pistoria, William D. Freeman.
    p. ; cm.
ISBN 978-0-19-996963-0 (alk. paper)
I. Josephson, Scott Andrew, author.   II. Pistoria, Michael Joseph, author.   III. Freeman, William
D., author.   IV. Title.
[DNLM: 1.   Central Nervous System Diseases—diagnosis—Handbooks.   2.   Hospitalists—
Handbooks.   3.   Neurologic Examination—Handbooks.   4.   Neurologic Manifestations—
Handbooks. WL 39]
RC348
616.8'0475—dc23
2013026662

The science of medicine is a rapidly changing field. As new research and clinical experience broaden our
knowledge, changes in treatment and drug therapy occur. The author and publisher of this work have
checked with sources believed to be reliable in their efforts to provide information that is accurate and
complete, and in accordance with the standards accepted at the time of publication. However, in light
of the possibility of human error or changes in the practice of medicine, neither the author, nor the
publisher, nor any other party who has been involved in the preparation or publication of this work
warrants that the information contained herein is in every respect accurate or complete. Readers are
encouraged to confirm the information contained herein with other reliable sources, and are strongly
advised to check the product information sheet provided by the pharmaceutical company for each drug
they plan to administer.

9 8 7 6 5 4 3 2 1
Printed in the United States of America
on acid-free paper

Dedication

Likosky: With love to my family: Laurin, Keely and Zane.
Josephson: Thanks to my loving family for their support.
Pistoria: To Angie, Maddie, Giana and Drew—you are my world.
Freeman: To my wife Michelle and daughter Lauren –je vous aime.

Contents

Foreword

Since the birth of the hospitalist movement, hospitalists have sought to define their scope of practice. This has evolved over time and there is significant variation nationally. Hospitalists frequently feel unprepared for the neurologic care they are expected to provide once in practice.

This handbook is written with that hospitalist in mind—a concise, practical guide to inpatient neurology care. We have presented a uniquely focused resource, not meant to replace textbooks, but rather to provide just what the practicing clinician needs to deliver excellent care to the individual and population of patients they see. Each chapter includes hospitalist and systems-specific categories such as proposed quality metrics and transitions of care considerations. This view of inpatient care will be of value likewise to medical students and residents as they manage patients with neurological signs, symptoms and diseases.

We hope, as hospitalists, neurologists and neurohospitalists that you find this handbook gives you the tools you need as you care for your patients.

1

Overview of Neuroanatomy

Introduction

A basic knowledge of neuroanatomy is a key component of the care of inpatients with neurologic problems. The ability to correlate signs on the neurologic examination with anatomy drives the selection of appropriate diagnostic tests and leads to effective diagnosis and treatment

1. Language Dysfunction (Aphasia)
    a. A focal sign localizing to the dominant hemisphere (the left hemisphere in nearly all right-handed individuals and also in the majority of those who are left-handed)
    b. Expressive (Broca's) aphasia: Difficulty with fluency but normal comprehension
        i. Patients are usually frustrated and can recognize their deficit
        ii. Inferior frontal lobe injury in the dominant hemisphere
    c. Receptive (Wernicke's) aphasia: Fluency preserved but comprehension impaired
        i. Patients often produce voluminous language which makes no sense and may not recognize their own deficits
        ii. Superior temporal lobe injury in the dominant hemisphere
    d. Global aphasia: Fluency and comprehension both impaired
        i. A larger area in the dominant hemisphere involving both Broca's and Wernicke's areas

2. Slurred Speech (dysarthria)
   a. The inability to pronounce words clearly
   b. Caused by injury to cranial nerves VII, X, or XII rather than injury to the areas of the homunculus in the brain corresponding to the mouth, tongue, or pharynx
3. Visual Loss
   a. Monocular visual loss indicates a lesion anterior to the optic chiasm either in the optic nerve or the eye itself
   b. Binocular visual loss is characteristic of damage to the visual pathways in the brain (Figure 1.1)
4. Double Vision
   a. Typically results when the eyes are not properly "yoked," suggesting dysfunction most commonly of the cranial nerves that control the eye (III, IV, VI) or, less commonly, the thalamus or midline cerebellum
   b. Double vision should resolve when either eye is covered
      i. Monocular double vision in contrast indicates either an ocular problem or is psychogenic
5. Weakness
   a. True neurologic weakness should be distinguished from that associated with pain, fatigue, or poor effort
   b. Weakness can result from injury to any part of the neuroaxis from the brain to the peripheral muscle
   c. The first step in evaluating a patient with weakness is localizing the problem as either an upper motor neuron (brain or spinal cord) or lower motor neuron (anterior horn cell, nerve, neuromuscular junction, or muscle) deficit (Table 1.1)
      i. The classic upper motor neuron signs of increased tone and reflexes may not be present acutely and will develop hours to days after the injury
   d. If the patient has upper motor neuron weakness, imaging of the brain or spinal cord is usually the next step in workup
      i. Clues to brain localization
         1. Aphasia
         2. Visual field deficit

3. Unilateral weakness or numbness, especially when involving the face
4. In the brainstem, the patient may have "crossed signs" with a cranial nerve deficit on one side of the body and weakness on the other

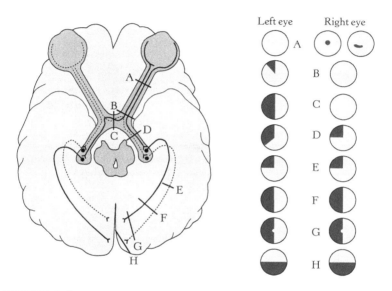

FIGURE 1.1

Patterns of visual field loss due to lesions at different locations along the visual pathway: A, optic nerve lesions result in a central scotoma or arcuate defect; B, optic nerve lesions just before the chiasma produce a junctional scotoma due to ipsilateral optic nerve involvement with the inferior contralateral crossing fibres (dashed lines); C, chiasmal lesions produce bitemporal hemianopia; D, optic tract lesions result in incongruous hemianopic defects; E, F lesions of the optic radiation result in either homonymous quadrantanopia or hemianopia depending on the extent and location of the lesion (upper quadrant, temporal lobe; lower quadrant, parietal lobe); G, lesions of the striate cortex produce a homonymous hemianopia, sometimes with macular sparing, particularly with vascular disturbances; H, lesions of the superior or inferior bank of the striate cortex result in inferior or superior altitudinal defects, respectively.

TABLE 1.1 Upper and Lower Motor Neuron Patterns of Weakness

	Upper Motor Neuron	*Lower Motor Neuron*
Pattern of weakness	Pyramidal*	Variable
Function/Dexterity	Slow alternating movements	Variable
Tone	Increased	Decreased
Tendon Reflexes	Increased	Decreased, absent or normal
Other signs	Babinski sign, other CNS signs	Atrophy (except for neuromuscular junction disorders)

*pyramidal: pattern of weakness characterized by increased weakness in distal muscles compared with proximal muscles as well as extensors>flexors in the upper extremities, and flexors>extensors in the lower extremities

  ii. Clues to spinal cord localization
    1. Paraparesis of the legs or quadriparesis (the latter can occur with brainstem injury as well)
    2. Bladder and/or bowel dysfunction
    3. Sensory level on the trunk
  e. If the patient has lower motor neuron weakness, imaging studies are generally not indicated, although electromyography/nerve conduction studies may allow for localization between anterior horn cell, nerve, neuromuscular junction, and muscle
    i. Clues to anterior horn cell localization
      1. Typically fasciculations are prominent
      2. A mixture of upper and lower motor neuron signs may accompany amyotrophic lateral sclerosis (ALS)

    ii. Clues to nerve localization

        1. The only lower motor neuron localization that features any sensory deficits

        2. May be in the distribution of a single peripheral nerve or nerve root rather than a more diffuse length-dependent polyneuropathy

        3. Reflexes are typically absent in the affected limbs

    iii. Clues to neuromuscular junction localization

        1. Weakness that fatigues or fluctuates over time or with repeated muscle testing

        2. Proximal > distal weakness common

    iv. Clues to muscle localization

        1. Proximal > distal weakness common

6. Sensory loss

    a. A difficult complaint to evaluate given the subjective nature of testing

    b. Large fiber nerves mediate vibration and joint position sense (proprioception) and connect with the dorsal column pathway in the spinal cord

    c. Small fiber nerves mediate pain and temperature and connect with the spinothalamic tract in the spinal cord

    d. Both systems then involve the thalamus and, finally, the contralateral cerebral cortex

    e. Clues to sensory localization (Figure 1.2)

        i. A pattern in the distribution of a single dermatome is usually a spinal root problem

        ii. A pattern in the distribution of a single nerve is usually a mononeuropathy

        iii. A sensory level on the trunk below which sensation is diminished typically is caused by a lesion in the spinal cord

7. Ataxia

    a. Typically caused by damage to the ipsilateral cerebellum or cerebellar connections in the brainstem or upper spinal cord

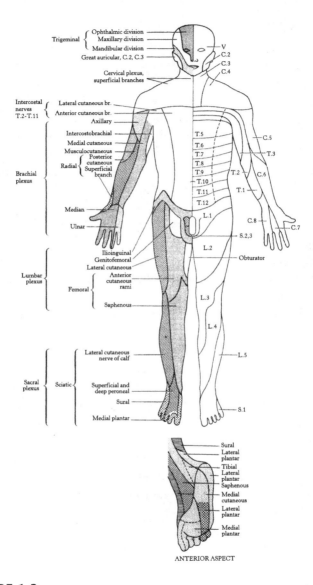

ANTERIOR ASPECT

FIGURE 1.2

Visual Localization

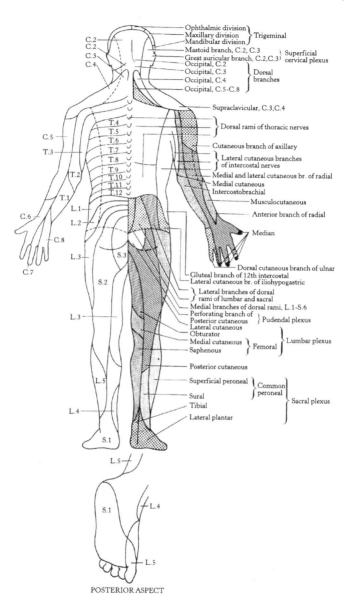

POSTERIOR ASPECT

FIGURE 1.2 (Continued)

    b. Sensory deficits can mimic this appearance (so-called "sensory ataxia")

    c. Cerebellar hemispheres can be tested with finger-nose-finger or heel-knee-shin

       i. Asymmetry indicates a structural lesion; symmetry usually indicates a metabolic etiology (e.g. drug intoxication)

    d. The midline cerebellar vermis is tested by watching the patient walk

       i. A wide-based unsteady gait is characteristic

2

History and Physical

Questions to Ask

1. When did the symptoms begin?
2. Were they sudden in onset or more insidious in nature?
3. Are there associated signs and symptoms?
4. Were there any prodromal symptoms?
5. You can begin parts of the neurologic evaluation while interviewing the patient
   a. Mental status and speech
      i. Is the patient paying appropriate attention to the interview?
      ii. Are they able to quickly and appropriately form answers to your questions?
      iii. Are there any abnormalities of speech?
      iv. What is the patient's mood?
   b. Cranial nerves
      i. Many can be evaluated during conversation
   c. Motor
      i. Is the patient sitting or lying down?
      ii. Note any asymmetries in movement
      iii. An externally rotated leg/ankle is a clue to weakness on that side
   d. Coordination
      i. As the patient reaches for things, touches their face, etc
      ii. Carefully watch the patient as they walk into the room or change positions

Key Pieces of the Neurological Evaluation

1. A routine neurological examination should focus on the following areas:
   a. Mental status
      i. Ask specific questions
   b. Cranial nerves
   c. Motor strength
      i. This should include fine motor function
   d. Reflexes
   e. Sensation
   f. Coordination
2. Depending upon the findings on the global neurologic examination, further attention should be paid to the specific areas
   a. Mental status
      i. Assess the patient's level of consciousness
      ii. Is the patient able to pay attention and concentrate on specific tasks?
      iii. How is the patient's short- and long-term memory
         1. Formally test with 1- and 3-minute three object recall
      iv. Speech
         1. Naming
         2. Ability to follow two-step commands
         3. take care not to perform the task you are asking for yourself; patients may mimic without understanding
      v. Higher-level cognition
         1. Consider full mini-mental status examination
         2. Serial sevens
         3. Ask patient to alternate alphabet and counting (a1, b2, c3)
      vi. Mood

b. Cranial nerves
    i. Note that olfaction is difficult to assess and is rarely tested
    ii. Cranial nerves II, III, VI, and VI
        1. Visual field testing
        2. Pupillary light reflex
        3. Eye movements
        4. Visual acuity
    iii. Cranial nerve V
        1. Symmetric facial sensation
        2. Corneal sensation
    iv. Cranial nerve VII
        1. Facial symmetry
        2. Upper motor neuron pattern spares forehead (MCA stroke)
        3. Lower motor neuron pattern includes forehead (Bell's Palsy)
    v. Cranial Nerve VIII
        1. Rub fingers together near patient's ears
    vi. Cranial nerve VIII
        1. Gait and balance
    vii. Cranial nerve IX and X
        1. Symmetric palate elevation
    viii. Cranial Nerve IX, X and XII
        1. Speech abnormalities a clue to dysfunction
    ix. Cranial nerve XII
        1. Head turning/shoulder shrug
    x. Cranial nerve XII
        1. Midline tongue protrusion
        2. Facial asymmetry is a potential confounder
c. Strength (overlaps with coordination)
    i. Observe the patient's gait
        1. Have the patient walk on their heels, on their toes, and do tandem walking

    ii. Assess coordination by having the patient do rapid alternating movements, finger-nose-finger and heel-to-shin testing

    iii. Pronator drift

        1. A sign of subtle weakness

        2. Look for true pronation

    iv. Test individual muscles by having the patient resist your attempts to move a given limb

        1. Medical Research Scale (MRS)

            a. 0—no strength

            b. 1—muscle movement only

            c. 2—able to move limb with gravity removed (parallel to floor)

            d. 3—able to move against gravity

            e. 4—< full strength

            f. 5—full strength

        2. Myotome map (Figure 2.1)

            a. Allows one to clarify muscle/nerve/nerve root involved

    v. Evaluate tone

        1. Rigidity as a sign of upper motor neuron damage

        2. Wasting as a sign of longstanding weakness

        3. Tremor

        4. Cogwheeling (as in Parkinson's disease)

d. Sensation (Figure 2.2)

    i. Is the patient able to identify light touch on the hands and feet?

    ii. Test the patient for symmetry in sensing *either* pain or temperature

    iii. Use a tuning fork to assess vibratory sense

    iv. Assess for graphesthesia, stereognosis, and two-point discrimination when indicated

e. Reflexes

    i. Allows definition of root level involved (Figure 2.3)

Muscle*	Roots	Nerve	Action
Trapezius	C3, 4	Spinal accessory	Shrug shoulder
Rhomboids	C4, 5	Dorsal scapular	Brace shoulders back
Supraspinatus	C5, 6	Suprascapular	Abduct shoulder 15°
Deltoid	C5, 6	Axillary	Abduct shoulder 15–90°
Infraspinatus of arm	C5, 6	Suprascapular	External rotation
Biceps	C5, 6	Musculocutaneous	Flex forearm
Triceps	C6, 7	Radial	Extend forearm
Extensor carpi	C5, 6	Radial	Extend wrist
Finger extensors	C7, 8	Posterior interosseous	Extend fingers
FDP I and II	C8, T1	Median	Flex DIPJ
FDP III and IV	C8, T1	Ulnar	Flex DIPJ
FDS	C8, T1	Median	Flex PIPJ
APB	C8, T1	Median	Abduct thumb
OP	C8, T1	Median	Thumb to 5th finger
ADM	C8, T1	Ulnar	Abduct 5th finger
1ST DIO	C8, T1	Ulnar	Abduct index finger
Iliopsoas	L1, 2	Femoral	Flex hip
Hip adductors	L2, 3	Obturator	Adduct hip
Hip extensors	L5, S1	Inferior gluteal	Extend hip
Quadriceps	L2, 3	Femoral	Extend knee
Hamstrings	L5, S1	Sciatic	Flex knee
Tibialis anterior	L5, S1	Deep peroneal	Dorsiflex foot
Gastrocnemius	S1, 2	Tibial	Plantarflex foot
Tibialis posterior	L4, 5	Tibial	Invert foot
EHL	L5, S1	Deep peroneal	Dorsiflex hallux
Peroneus longus	L5, S1	Superficial peroneal	Evert foot

*Muscles in bold font are essential in a basic neurological examination.

FIGURE 2.1

Important myotomes

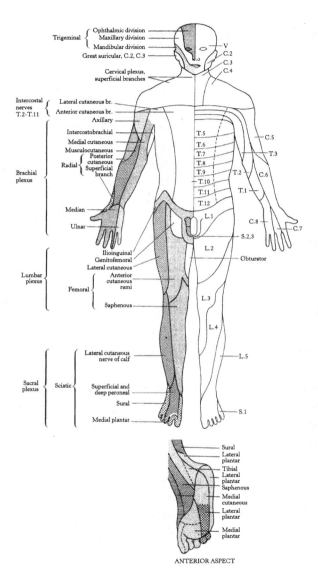

FIGURE 2.2

Dermatomes

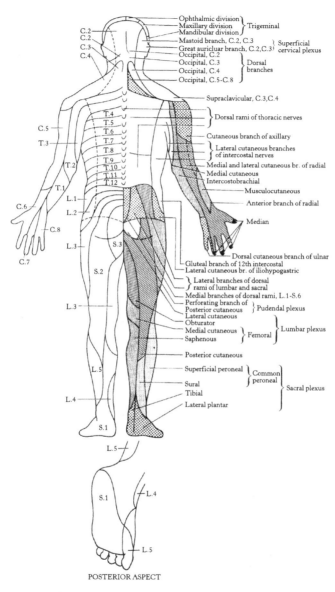

Ophthalmic division ⎫
Maxillary division ⎬ Trigeminal
Mandibular division ⎭
Mastoid branch, C.2, C.3
Great auricluar branch, C.2,C.3 ⎫ Superficial
Occipital, C.2 ⎭ cervical plexus
Occipital, C.3 ⎫
Occipital, C.4 ⎬ Dorsal branches
Occipital, C.5-C.8 ⎭

Supraclavicular, C.3,C.4

Dorsal rami of thoracic nerves

Cutaneous branch of axillary

Lateral cutaneous branches of intercostal nerves

Medial and lateral cutaneous br. of radial
Medial cutaneous
Intercostobrachial
Musculocutaneous
Anterior branch of radial
Median

Dorsal cutaneous branch of ulnar
Gluteal branch of 12th intercostal
Lateral cutaneous br. of iliohypogastric
Lateral branches of dorsal rami of lumbar and sacral
Medial branches of dorsal rami, L.1-S.6
Perforating branch of ⎫
Posterior cutaneous ⎬ Pudendal plexus
Lateral cutaneous
Obturator
Medial cutaneous ⎫ Femoral ⎫ Lumbar plexus
Saphenous ⎭

Posterior cutaneous

Superficial peroneal ⎫ Common
Sural peroneal ⎭ Sacral plexus
Tibial
Lateral plantar

POSTERIOR ASPECT

FIGURE 2.2 (Continued)

Reflex	Nerve	Root
Biceps	Musculocutaneous	C5/6
Supinator	Radial	C5/6
Triceps	Radial	C7
Finger flexors	Median/ulnar	C8
Knee	Femoral	L3/4
Ankle	Tibial	S1/2

FIGURE 2.3

Deep tendon reflexes

    ii. It is very helpful to distract the patient while doing reflex testing

    iii. Remember that it is most important to compare reflexes between sides

    iv. Grading

        1. 0—no response

        2. 1—trace response

        3. 2—normal response

        4. 3—hyperactive response

        5. 4—sustained clonus

    v. Isometric effort may accentuate difficult to elicit reflexes

3

Stroke Overview/Pathophysiology

Questions to Ask

1. What type of stroke was it?
    i. 85% of all strokes occur from blockage of an artery (ischemic) which reduces cerebral blood flow (CBF) to an intracranial artery vascular territory (Figure 3.1)
        1. Main vascular divisions
            a. The anterior circulation
                i. internal carotid artery (ICA) divides into the anterior cerebral artery (ACA) and middle cerebral artery (MCA)
            b. The posterior circulation
                i. Paired vertebral arteries feed the singular basilar artery which ends in the posterior cerebral arteries (PCA)
            c. The circle of Willis is present in 15% of individuals who have vascular collaterals between MCA, ACA, PCA circulations (Figure 3.2)
        2. Clinical syndromes depend on the functional neuroanatomic brain tissue affected
        3. Small vessel disease (branches of the main intracranial vessels mentioned above) typically causes hypodensity of the white matter (leukoariosis) on CT and small discrete lacunar infarctions within the deep basal ganglia or deep locations

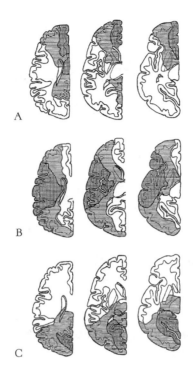

FIGURE 3.1

Cerebral arterial territories. Horizontal sections of the brain to show areas supplied by the anterior (A), middle (B), and posterior (C) cerebral arteries. The vertical lines represent the smallest and the horizontal lines the largest areas of supply in various individuals. (With permission from Dr Albert van der Zwan, University of Utrecht.)

      4. Watershed (borderzone) ischemia occurs from either hypotension or profound anemia (or both) and sometimes with vascular stenotic/occlusive disease. The borderzone area is the region between 2 vascular territories

  ii. 15% of all strokes are hemorrhagic

      1. Intraparenchymal hematoma (IPH) or intracerebral hemorrhage (ICH) –bleeding typically from submillimeter

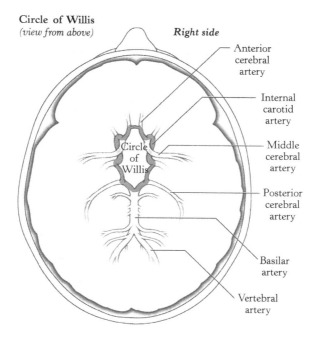

Circle of Willis
(view from above)   *Right side*

- Anterior cerebral artery
- Internal carotid artery
- Middle cerebral artery
- Posterior cerebral artery
- Basilar artery
- Vertebral artery

Circle of Willis

FIGURE 3.2

Circle of Willis. Used with permission of Mayo Foundation for Medical Education and Research, all rights reserved.

   parenchymal   perforators   usually   from   chronic hypertension
2. Typical locations include the putamen, thalamus, cerebellum, and pons
3. Other etiologies include trauma and underlying abnormalities such as tumors, infection, and arteriovenous malformation (AVMs)
4. Cerebral amyloid angiopathy (CAA) is a fragile blood vessel condition in the elderly that can cause ICH, often in cortical/lobar locations (Figure 3.3)

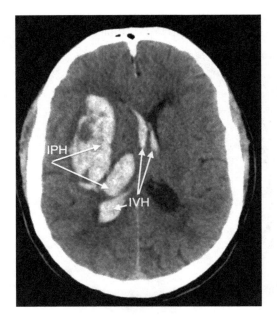

FIGURE 3.3

Intracranial Hemorrhage. IVH = intraventricular hemorrhage.
IPH = Intraparenchymal hemorrhage

> 5. Subarachnoid hemorrhage (SAH) is caused most commonly by trauma or rupture of an intracranial aneurysm around the Circle of Willis which creates a characteristic pattern on CT (Figure 3.4)
>
> 2. What is normal cerebrovascular physiology?
>   a. CPP = MAP − ICP, where MAP = mean arterial pressure, ICP = intracranial pressure (in mmHg)
>   b. Autoregulation indicates that CBF is held constant across a varying range of CPP due to changes in CVR (cerebral vessel reactivity) (Figure 3.5)

3. What is abnormal stroke pathophysiology?
   a. Cushing's reflex—a protective brain reflex which increases blood pressure), and causes bradycardia when ICP is elevated. Typically lessens over 24–48hrs or if ICP or brain insult is removed
   b. In stroke, the injured brain tissue loses its ability to autoregulate and becomes "pressure passive" reacting directly to pressure changes rather than plateauing, as in Figure 3.5; instead of a horizontal line, the relationship becomes linear up sloping
   c. Core region of brain tissue infarction is an area of brain tissue that is destined for infarction within minutes unless CBF is reestablished immediately

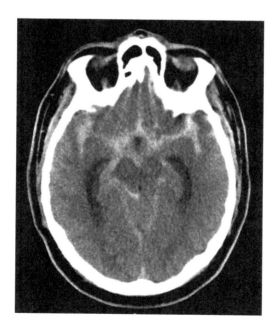

FIGURE 3.4

Subarachnoid Hemorrhage

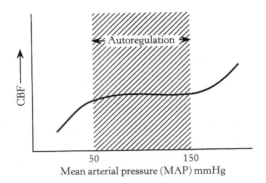

FIGURE 3.5

A diagram to illustrate autoregulation of cerebral blood flow (CBF) in normal man. Between a mean arterial blood pressure (MAP) of about 50–150mmHg, CBF remains roughly constant. Reprinted with permission of Rothwell P, Brain's Diseases of the Nervous System: Cerebrovascular Diseases. Oxford University Press.

    d. Penumbra is a regional of potentially salvageable brain tissue that has borderline blood flow and can be saved if blood flow is established in a timely fashion. Acute stroke therapies are meant to target this region

Diagnostic Tests

1. Imaging relating to pathophysiology
   a. Noncontrast head CT is the test used to distinguish between ischemic stroke, and hemorrhagic stroke with >98% sensitivity
   b. MRI has takes more time but can distinguish as well
   c. MRI is more sensitive to ischemia and infarction, especially early
   d. Ischemic stroke within several hours of onset may show only "early ischemic signs" (Figure 3.6)

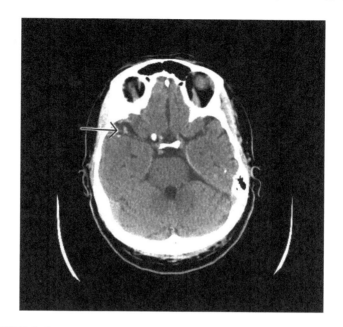

FIGURE 3.6

Early Signs of Ischemia and stroke. Dense middle cerebral artery (clot) sign shown (arrow). Used with permission of Mayo Foundation for Medical Education and Research, all rights reserved.

     i. Early sulci/gyri effacement or edema seen around the Sylvian fissure compared to the contralateral side: "insular ribbon sign"
    ii. May portend
       1. Worse overall outcome
       2. Higher NIH stroke scale severity (NIH)
       3. Lesser chance of recanalization with IV-tPA

Management Considerations

1. Acute blood pressure management (Figure 3.7)

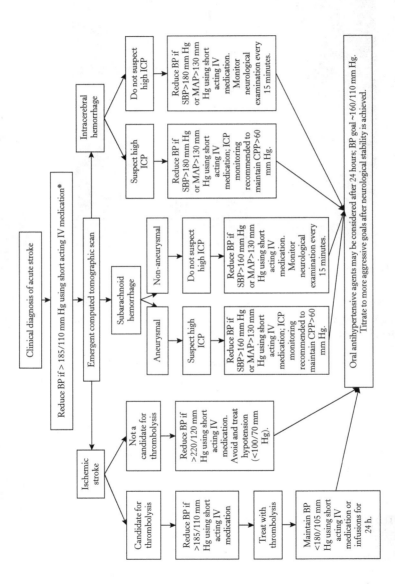

FIGURE 3.7

Blood Pressure Management in Stroke. Modified and permission granted from Qureshi AI. Circulation 2008; 118: 176-187

a. Ischemic stroke management is typically predicated on "permissive hypertension" to allow perfusion of CBF to areas of surrounding brain that are at risk of infarction

b. Hemorrhagic stroke is different than ischemic stroke because high blood pressure can lead to further intracranial bleeding. As a result, blood pressure is typically controlled rather than allowing permissive hypertension

2. Reperfusion injury

   a. A concern when an area has had decreased blood flow which is then restored

   b. May be seen post carotid revascularization

   c. Results in edema and potential for hemorrhagic conversion

4

TIA Evaluation

Questions to Ask

1. Was it a TIA?
   a. Assess for potential risk factors
   b. The more significant the symptoms, the simpler to diagnose
   c. Interview witnesses if possible
   d. Elements of the ABCD² score (below) helpful
2. Does the patient need to be admitted?
   a. Ideal to set up criteria ahead of time, in agreement with neurology, emergency department
   b. Little data on efficacy of admission
   c. Strongly consider when to followup an issue
   d. Strongly consider when patient is at very high risk of short-term stroke (see ABCD² scoring)
3. What is the difference between time-based and tissue-based definitions for TIA?
   a. Time-based is the traditional definition (symptoms lasting < 24 hours with complete resolution)
   b. Tissue-based approaches are becoming more common
      i. Even with symptom resolution, there is frequently evidence of a new infarction (up to 30–40%)
      ii. No evidence of infarction on imaging (typically MRI) defines a TIA
      iii. Argues for treating TIA in the same way you treat stroke
4. What is the likelihood the patient will have a stroke?
   a. Risk as high as 10% in 90 days

Criteria	Point system
A Age	1
B Blood pressure ≥140/90 mmHg	1 point for hypertension at the acute evaluation
C Clinical features	2 points for unilateral weakness, 1 for speech disturbance without weakness
D Symptom Duration	1 point for 10–59 min, 2 points for ≥60 min
D Diabetes	1 point

FIGURE 4.1

The ABCD2 tool for transient ischaemic attack

    b. ABCD^2 score helps predict risk but alternate systems may be more accurate and useful (Figure 4.1)
       i. 2 day stroke risk based on score
          1. 0–3: 1%
          2. 4–5: 4.1%
          3. 6–7: 8.1%
    c. ABCD^3 score adds 2 points for a TIA within 7days prior to the index TIA
    d. ABCD^3-I adds 2 points for ≥50% carotid stenosis and 2 points for a diffusion weighted imaging abnormality on MRI (indicative of acute ischemia)
    5. What is a RIND?
       a. Reversible ischemic deficit—old terminology that is not clinically useful

Exam Findings

    1. Typically, symptoms will have resolved
    2. A careful neurological exam essential to find any residual deficits

Diagnostic Tests

1. Imaging
   a. May reveal prior or acute infarcts
      i. Old infarcts indicate increased risk for future strokes
   b. CT
      i. Insensitive for acute ischemia, but can exclude mimics (e.g. a tumor or subdural hematoma leading to seizures)
   c. MRI
      i. May show evidence of acute ischemia or infarct for which symptoms have resolved
      ii. Being used increasingly in setting of TIA
   d. Carotid evaluation
      i. Should be performed in an expedited fashion
      ii. With ultrasound or CTA/MRA
2. Labs
   a. As per ischemic stroke evaluation
      i. CBC, BMP, PT/PTT, fasting lipid panel
      ii. Further laboratory evaluation for patients without traditional risk factors
3. Echocardiography
   a. Routinely recommended
   b. If high index of suspicion for PFO/structural abnormality or large habitus, consider transesophageal exam
4. Arrhythmia monitoring
   a. Multiple potential approaches (see idiopathic stroke chapter)
   b. Consider in setting of high probability TIA diagnosis and potential for arrhythmia or lack of traditional risk factors
5. EEG—rarely indicated unless high index of suspicion for seizure

Treatment Options

1. Similar to that of ischemic stroke—see ischemic stroke chapter for more detail
2. Antiplatelet agent should be started or changed
3. Anti-hypertensives should be started with a goal of good control
4. Strongly consider starting a statin pending lipid results

When to Consider Consulting a Neurologist

1. Uncertain diagnosis
2. Uncertain next steps for therapy or imaging evaluation
3. To help assure close follow-up

Care Transitions

1. Close follow-up essential given high short term risk of completed stroke

Proposed Quality Metrics

1. Initiation of appropriate secondary prevention
2. Assurance of appropriate follow-up
3. Documentation of risk stratification score

Ischemic Stroke

Questions to Ask

1. Is it really a stroke?
   a. Important to keep a differential diagnosis in mind, especially when aggressive therapies are being considered
   b. Imaging is very helpful, but stroke is still a clinical diagnosis
2. Is the stroke hemorrhagic or ischemic?
   a. The biggest branch point in care
   b. Can not reliably tell by physical examination
   c. Most rapid determination by CT
   d. CT and MRI have similar sensitivity
3. Is the patient a candidate for aggressive intervention?
   a. Thrombolysis both intravenous and intra-arterial as well as mechanical retrieval increasingly are being used
   b. Important to consider as early as possible
   c. Approach each patient as a potential candidate until proven otherwise
4. Does your hospital have a stroke system in place?
   a. Joint Commission Disease Specific Certification is one path to achieving a uniform process of care
   b. Process-of-care measures are critical to rapid treatment
      i. Rapid triage
      ii. Laboratory draws +/- point-of-care testing
      iii. Imaging, expedited scanning, and interpretation
      iv. Ability to mix and deliver tPA quickly when needed

   c. Nurse training is critical
     i. Focused neurological exam, standardized
     ii. Awareness of potential complications and when to call
   d. Physician communication is critical
     i. Consider conferences for case reviews
     ii. Consider National Institutes of Health Stroke Scale (NIHSS) certification for emergency physicians, hospitalists, and neurologists

Exam Findings

1. Given the implications of posterior circulation stroke, important to be aware of those findings
   a. Posterior circulation refers to the area of the brain served by the vertebrobasilar system; includes the brainstem and cerebellum
   b. Anterior circulation fed by the internal carotid arteries
   c. Cranial nerve findings a hallmark of posterior fossa lesions
     i. Diplopia
     ii. Nystagmus, especially vertical
     iii. Anisocoria or unequal pupils (may indicate elevated intracranial pressure as well)
     iv. Perioral numbness
2. Pattern recognition key
   a. Vascular distributions result in characteristic deficits
   b. Middle cerebral artery strokes tend to be best recognized
     i. Dominant hemisphere with speech deficit and weakness/numbness on contralateral side
     ii. Nondominant similar without speech deficit, but commonly with perceptual deficits/apraxia (inability to perform a task despite the understanding/strength to do so)

    c. Anterior cerebral artery strokes less common
      i. Foot/leg weakness and sensory loss
      ii. Apraxia
      iii. Abulia (lack of will/initiative)
    d. Posterior cerebral artery strokes
      i. Visual field deficits most common
3. Careful neurological exam should be performed on all patients and documented
    a. Documentation key to other providers being able to assess for changes in status

Diagnostic Tests

1. Imaging
    a. Emergent imaging assesses for presence of blood, alternate diagnoses, prior strokes, and early changes
    b. CT
      i. Insensitive for acute ischemia
      ii. Similar sensitivity to MRI for acute hemorrhage
      iii. The most rapid test
      iv. Contrast typically unnecessary unless looking at vasculature
      v. A bright (or hyperdense) artery sign may indicate clot in major blood vessel
        1. Increased risk for malignant MCA infarction (>1/3 of MCA territory) with edema and worse outcome
    c. CT angiography
      i. Requires contrast and good IV access
      ii. Many centers use as part of their acute stroke evaluation
      iii. Allows rapid evaluation of anterior and posterior circulation
      iv. Rapid evaluation for thrombus, dissection, stenosis
      v. Risks with impaired GFR

    d. MRI

        i. Most sensitive to acute ischemia/infarction

        ii. May delay therapy unless systems set up to expedite scans

    e. MR angiography

        i. Provides a good view of vasculature

        ii. Requires access

        iii. Risks with impaired GFR

    f. Carotid ultrasound

        i. User dependent, but rapid

        ii. May be unnecessary if angiography being performed

    g. Conventional angiography

        i. Seldom used in stroke unless patient undergoing mechanical thrombectomy or intraarterial thrombolysis

        ii. In cases of concern for vasculitis

            1. Typically presents with multiple strokes and inflammatory CSF

            2. Associated with confusion

            3. May be isolated, i.e. not a part of a systemic vasculitis

2. Labs

    a. Important to expedite so that contrast can be given if appropriate and aggressive therapies including tPA used

        i. CBC

            1. Rule out thrombocytopenia

            2. Rule out hematologic abnormalities that might preclude therapies or interfere with oxygen delivery

        ii. BMP/Chem7

            1. Creatinine important for contrast studies

            2. Electrolyte abnormalities may explain neurologic abnormalities

        iii. Glucose level

            1. May explain neurologic symptoms

            2. May diagnose previously unknown diabetes

        iv. PT/PTT

            1. Screen for anticoagulant use

2. Evaluate eligibility for thrombolytics (INR≤ 1.7 for tPA given 0–3 hours from last seen normal)
3. May be helpful in identifying underlying coagulopathy
4. Note newer anticoagulants have variable effects and a careful medication history is essential

v. Fasting lipid panel
1. Indicated for all stroke patients
2. Helps establish baseline for outpatient follow-up

vi. Hemoglobin A1c
1. May be useful to screen for diabetes

vii. Further laboratory evaluation for patients without traditional risk factors

3. Echocardiography
a. Routinely recommended without clear criteria for select populations in whom it may have higher yield
b. Important to order when it would affect your management
c. May be a clue to arrhythmia
d. If high index of suspicion for patent foramen ovale/structural abnormality or large habitus consider transesophageal exam

4. Arrhythmia monitoring
a. Routinely performed during inpatient stay while on telemetry unit
b. Outpatient follow-up monitoring may be performed for brief (48 hours) to extended (30 days or greater) periods of time
c. Event monitors may be useful if patient is symptomatic

5. EEG—rarely indicated unless high index of suspicion for seizure

Treatment Options

1. Best to initiate secondary prevention therapy in the hospital when possible—this has been shown to increase compliance

2. Antiplatelet agents
    a. Aspirin
        i. Significant difference in morbidity, mortality and recurrent stroke rates
        ii. No significant differences in doses
        iii. Lowest cost
    b. Clopidogrel
        i. Marginal benefit over aspirin
        ii. Has potential cardiovascular benefit as well
        iii. Once daily
    c. Aspirin-Dipyridamole
        i. Marginal benefit over aspirin
        ii. Twice daily
        iii. Headache a potential side effect
    d. Dual anti-platelet therapy (clopidogrel and aspirin)
        i. Subject of ongoing study, especially in minor stroke
3. Anticoagulants
    a. Heparin
        i. Very limited utility in acute stroke
        ii. Consider in dissection, venous thrombosis, intracardiac clot
        iii. If used, consider avoiding boluses and supratherapeutic PTT, which raise risk of hemorrhage
    b. Warfarin or newer anticoagulants (direct thrombin or factor Xa inhibitors)
        i. Indicated in cases of arrhythmia, coagulopathy
4. Anti-hypertensives
    a. Typically started at low dose subacutely
    b. Permissive hypertension, i.e. allowing bp 220/120 in the acute period is commonly recommended per international guidelines without high quality data
    c. When medications are used acutely
        i. start in low doses and titrate as needed
        ii. Intravenous beta blockers and nicardipine commonly used

    d. Consider other comorbidities (e.g., ace inhibitors for diabetics)

5. Statins
   a. Benefit even with normal lipids
   b. Some debate over role of high dose statins
   c. Do not increase risk of subsequent hemorrhage

6. tPA
   a. indicated for acute ischemic stroke with significant deficit and last seen normal 0–3 hours
   b. data also supports (some debate) its use to 4.5 hours from last seen normal with additional criteria
   c. important to recognize potential contraindications; see potential contraindications section
   d. Note blood pressure exclusions—SBP >185 mm Hg and DBP >110 mm Hg (if aggressive treatment required)
   e. ICU monitoring after administration
   f. Antiplatelet agents started 24 hours after tPA
   g. Intra-arterial tPA may be used up to 6 hours

7. Mechanical thrombectomy
   a. Up to 8 hours after time last seen normal; perhaps longer in basilar artery
   b. Dynamic area with ongoing improvement in devices
   c. Requires a specific clot in large vessel (target lesion)
   d. At present, data not as robust as that of tPA

8. Carotid revascularization
   a. Should be performed within a short period of time (<2 weeks) after non-disabling stroke

When to Consider Consulting a Neurologist

1. Uncertain diagnosis
2. Uncertain next steps for therapy or imaging evaluation
3. Ongoing management of risk factors/recovery
4. In cases of evident intracranial or extracranial stenosis

5. To help assure close follow-up

Care Transitions

1. Assure communication of neurological exam when moving between units and shifts
2. Sign outs important, especially in patients who have had lytic therapy or intervention and are at higher risk for hemorrhagic transformation/complications
3. Education prior to discharge
   a. Need to seek emergent care if recurrent stroke symptoms and what those symptoms are
   b. Medications and their purpose
   c. Patient-specific risk factors for stroke
   d. Need for outpatient follow-up
4. Blood pressure goals short-term (i.e., within 2 weeks) and long-term in outpatient setting, and communicated to patient, caregiver, and the outpatient physician or team

Other Considerations

1. Joint Commission stroke center certification provides a framework for standardizing care processes
2. Assure physical therapy and occupational therapy evaluate the patient
3. Assure a swallow screen is performed prior to any oral intake including medications. If there is any concern about swallowing, a formal swallow evaluation should be performed
4. Low threshold for inpatient or outpatient rehabilitation/ physiatry consultation
5. VTE prophylaxis critical given prevalence of impaired mobility

Special Clinical Situations

1. Posterior circulation stroke
   a. Includes vertebral/basilar circulation
   b. Longer time windows for intervention given the potentially grave outcomes
2. Intracranial stenosis
   a. At present no data that intervention better than aggressive medical management
   b. Antiplatelets as effective as anticoagulation in symptomatic stenosis with less risk of complications
3. Carotid stenosis
   a. Revascularize for symptomatic >70% stenosis if patients are at average or better risk and operator complications rates are <6%
   b. Subpopulations may benefit from either carotid artery stenting or carotid endarterectomy, referral to a vascular neurologist/skilled surgeon important
   c. Increasing data that medical management may be the best option in asymptomatic stenosis
4. Idiopathic stroke
   a. Stroke without traditional risk factors
   b. Expanded work-up (partial list)
      i. Coagulopathy
      ii. Angiography (MR, CT or conventional)
      iii. Arrhythmia monitoring (extended time period)
      iv. Transesophageal echocardiography
      v. Autoimmune/collagen vascular abnormalities
      vi. Infectious causes (syphilis)
      vii. EEG
   c. Neurology consultation

Proposed Quality Metrics

1. Process of care/timeliness measures for acute stroke evaluation
   a. Time to lab results
   b. Time to imaging read availability
2. Timeliness of treatment initiation for acute stroke
3. VTE prophylaxis
4. Dysphagia screening
5. Evaluation by physical and occupational therapy
6. Secondary prevention medication initiation
7. Education prior to discharge
8. Assurance of post-discharge follow-up
9. Minimal use of urinary catheters

Potential contraindications for tPA from 0–3 hours from last seen normal

- Younger than 18 years old
- Major surgery within 14 days
- Recent lumbar puncture
- Glucose below 50 or >400
- Platelet count <100,000
- INR > than 1.7
- Receiving oral anticoagulant *and* INR unknown or >1.7—or use of newer anticoagulants
- History of intracranial hemorrhage (aneurysm, AV malformation)
- Stroke in prior 3 months
- GI or GU hemorrhage within 21 days
- Myocardial infarction in prior 3 months
- Evidence of active bleeding or acute trauma (fracture)
- Head trauma in prior 3 months
- Symptoms improving/minor, NIHSS <4

- Receiving heparin, low molecular weight heparin, direct thrombin inhibitor, or factor Xa inhibitor within 48 hours *and* elevated PTT or elevated anti-Xa level
- Seizure with postictal residual neurological impairments
- SBP >185 mm Hg and DBP >110 mm Hg (if aggressive treatment required)

Additional contraindications for tPA from 3–4.5 hours from last seen normal

- Patient older than 80 years
- NIH stroke scale > 25
- Receiving oral anticoagulant (warfarin, direct thrombin inhibitor, factor Xa inhibitor)
- History of stroke and diabetes

6

Hemorrhagic Stroke

Questions to Ask

1. What type of intracranial hemorrhage (ICH) was it?
    i. Subarachnoid hemorrhage (SAH)—bleeding within the subarachnoid space. Typically has a classic "star" pattern around the basal cisterns (Figure 6.1) but those with less volume of blood may be more subtle
    ii. Intraparenchymal hematoma (IPH) or intracerebral hematoma (ICH)—bleeding within the brain parenchyma (Figure 6.2)
    iii. Intraventricular hematoma (IVH)—blood that is within the ventricles of the brain (Figure 6.2)
    iv. Subdural hematoma (SDH)—bleeding within the subdural space (Figure 6.3)
        1. typically has crescent appearance on CT scan
        2. does not respect cranial suture lines
    v. Epidural hematoma (EDH)—bleeding within the epidural space
        1. typically a lens or wedge shaped hematoma on CT scan
        2. respects suture lines
    vi. Traumatic ICH (tICH)—typically associated with a significant unprotected fall with closed head injury
2. Is the ICH due to an underlying vascular cause?
    a. Aneurysmal subarachnoid hemorrhage
        i. Ruptured cerebral aneurysm
        ii. Arteriovenous malformation
        iii. Other vascular anomaly

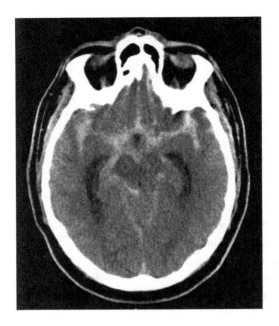

FIGURE 6.1

Subarachnoid Hemorrhage

> iv. typically has a "thunderclap" sudden onset of worst headache of one's life and/or neurologic deficit(s); headache typically reaches maximal intensity over seconds to minutes

a. Hypertensive intraparenchymal bleeding
   i. may have a sudden neurologic onset
   ii. typically located in deep parenchymal locations
      1. basal ganglia (putamen especially), thalamus, pons, cerebellum

b. Cerebral amyloid angiopathy (CAA)
   i. fragile blood vessel disorder seen with increasing age, especially those over 70
   ii. Pathology overlaps with Alzheimer disease

c. SDH and EDH are typically traumatic in origin, rarely vascular

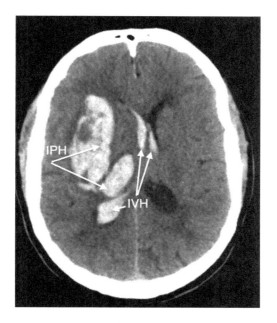

FIGURE 6.2

Intraparenchymal hemorrhage (IPH) with intraventricular hemorrhage (IVH) extension

Exam Findings

1. Physical examination
    a. Evidence of trauma:
        i. Cranial/facial/cervical trauma
            1. Raccoon's eyes (periorbital ecchymosis)
            2. Battles sign (ecchymosis behind the mastoid)
            3. Spinal step off or injury (palpable irregularity indicating fracture)
            4. Cephalohematoma (palpable blood under the periosteum)
            5. If any evidence of C-spine injury, immobilize the C-spine with a C-collar and consult appropriately

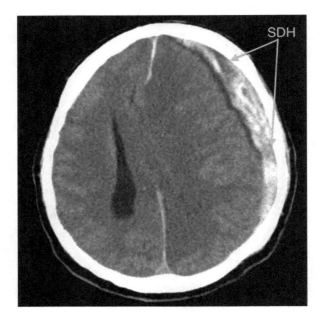

FIGURE 6.3

Subarachnoid hematoma, SDH

    b. Global neurologic assessment

        i. Consider intubation if Glasgow coma scale (GCS, Table 6.1) ≤8 via rapid sequence intubation protocol

  2. Neurologic severity

    a. NIH stroke scale

    b. Complete neurologic exam to document the neurologic deficits

  3. Physical examination including oral cavity, chest, abdomen, and extremities for findings of trauma

Diagnostic Tests

  1. Imaging

    a. Noncontrast head CT

TABLE 6.1 The Glasgow Coma Scale (Teasdale and Jennett 1974)

Eye-opening response
4 Spontaneous
3 To speech
2 To painful stimulus
1 None

Best motor response in upper limbs
6 Obeys commands
5 Localizes
4 Withdraws (normal flexion)
3 Flexes abnormally (spastic flexion)
2 Extends
1 None

Verbal response
5 Oriented
4 Confused
3 Inappropriate words
2 Incomprehensive sounds
1 None

Reprinted with permission of Donaghy M, Brain's Diseases of the Nervous System: Cerebrovascular Diseases. Oxford University Press.

    i. Most commonly used test
    ii. Extremely sensitive for intraparenchymal blood
    iii. Hemorrhage shows as bright/hyperdense (Figures 6.1–6.3)
    iv. For minor (sentinel) SAH bleeding, the CT scan sensitivity decreases with time for small leaks, that is, >95% detection day #1, ~75% day #2, 50% day #3 with further decreases further with time
  b. Contrast head CT
    i. May show evidence of ongoing bleeding—"spot sign" with higher morbidity and mortality
  c. Volume of blood correlates with mortality
    i. The volume of intraparenchymal bleeding can be estimated if elliptical by the ABC/2 formula in which A and B are the visually largest perpendicular diameters

(cm), and C is the vertical diameter which can be calculated by the number of slices in which the IPH is seen multiplied by slice thickness

    ii. One-month mortality ~ 30% with $30ml^3$ IPH and ~ 50% with >$45ml^3$

d. The blood pattern of ICH typically indicates the possible underlying pathology

    i. Spherical or ellipsoid bleeding within the parenchyma near the basal ganglia, pons, caudate or internal capsule is typically associated with "hypertensive" IPH and not aneurysmal

    ii. Intraparenchymal hemorrhage (IPH) near the cortical-subcortical locations in older patients is most commonly due to CAA

    iii. Star-shaped pattern near the basal cisterns is typically SAH which is usually aneurysmal or traumatic

    iv. Convex or lens shaped hematoma on the cortical convexity is typically EDH and stays between skull suture lines

    v. Crescent-shaped (like a quarter moon) which is beyond skull suture lines is typically SDH

e. Cerebral angiography

    i. If aneurysmal subarachnoid hemorrhage is suspected

    ii. Potential to treat with endovascular coiling versus open craniotomy and surgical clipping

f. MRI with contrast

    i. If unknown cause of bleeding

    ii. Gradient echo sequences may reveal CAA pathology, which appear as multiple tiny black dots typically in lobar (cortical-subcortical) locations

        1. Multiple tiny black dots in deep locations such as the basal ganglia, thalamus, capsule are suggestive of chronic hypertensive vasculopathy with microhemorrhages

2. Labs
   a. PT/INR and PTT
      i. In patients taking dabigatran, the aPTT correlates loosely with the level of anticoagulant effect. Thrombin Time (TT) and ecarin (ECT) correlate more closely with anticoagulant effect, but are not available or timely enough for clinical management. No known antidote is known for reversal of dabigatran, but the manufacturer recommends IV hydration to increase glomerular excretion of the drug, and in life-threating cases dialysis can remove the drug
   b. CBC with platelet count
   c. Pregnancy testing (urine testing can return quicker than serum in some labs) and before any X rays are performed.
   d. Fingerstick glucose to evaluate for glycemic control
   e. Urine or blood toxicology screening as appropriate if illicit drug use such as sympathomimetics, cocaine is suggested by the history

Treatment

1. Intraparenchymal and intraventricular hemorrhage
   a. intraparenchymal hemorrhage (IPH) extends through the parenchyma into the cerebrospinal fluid (CSF)-filled ventricles (Figure 6.2)
   b. can cause obstructive (blocking CSF ouflow) or non-obstructive (communicating) hydrocephalus
   c. may warrant neurosurgical placement of a external ventricular drain (EVD) or similar and for ICP monitoring, in patients felt to have a potential for recovery
   d. Acute blood pressure management (<2hrs) should be kept < 180 mmHg when ICP is felt not to be elevated. Randomized studies INTERACT and ATACH II underway targeting more

aggressive BP control (<140 systolic vs. 180) on hematoma expansion and clinical outcomes

2. Surgical evacuation of intraparenchymal hemorrhage

   a. Less commonly performed than in prior years due to large randomized study, especially deep IPH (PMID: Mendelow AD et al 15680453)

   b. Consider drainage

     i. Lobar, superficial bleeds in younger patients

     ii. Cerebellar hematoma 3cm or greater in size with symptomatic mass effect or obstructive hydrocephalus at the level of the cerebral aqueduct or 4th ventricle

   c. Studies of minimally invasive techniques underway

3. Subarachnoid hemorrhage

   a. Largely neurosurgical/interventional neuroradiology/neurocritical care driven to secure (coiling or clipping) of the aneurysm as soon as possible to prevent subsequent rebleeding. Exceptions may include moribund patients

   b. General trend toward endovascular approaches more than clipping based on available data

   c. Pre and post-operative care complex with considerations of blood pressure management, ICP monitoring if hydrocephalus is present, and vasospasm

   d. Acute blood pressure management (< 24hrs) should be kept < 140–160mmHg until aneurysm is secured unless ICP is elevated

4. Subdural/Epidural Hematoma

   a. Treatment largely surgical evacuation, especially for rapidly expanding hematomas, those 2cm or greater in maximal thickness and/or with symptomatic mass effect with neurological deficits

   b. Antiplatelets and anticoagulants can usually be started soon after surgery if indicated, important to discuss with neurosurgery/neurology in each case

5. Minimize complications
   a. avoid hypoxemia
   b. avoid hyperglycemia (> 180mg/dl)
   c. maintain adequate cerebral perfusion pressure (CPP >65) and ICP <20mmHg if monitored
   d. careful attention to dysphagia and aspiration risk
   e. venous thromboembolism prophylaxis with sequential compression devices initially and general avoidance of heparinoids for the first 24–48hrs until ICH is stabilized and if cleared by the neurosurgeon
6. Cerebral edema
   a. refer to chapter on elevated intracranial pressure
   b. treatment options include EVD and noninvasive treatments such as mannitol and hypertonic saline
7. Minimize further bleeding
   a. Antiplatelet therapy
      i. Hold for at least 48 hours (consider consult if recent stents)
      ii. Platelet transfusions debated, no clear evidence favoring
   b. Anticoagulation
      i. Normalize INR (INR < 1.5) if ICH/IPH/IVH/SDH on warfarin
      ii. Assure follow-up INR ordered after reversal agents given
      iii. Fresh frozen plasma (FFP) or prothrombin complex concentrate (PCC)
         1. No difference in outcome/mortality has been shown
         2. FFP involves more volume
         3. PCC reverses INR more rapidly
      iv. Intravenous vitamin K 10mg– low risk (1/10,000) of anaphylactic/anaphylactoid reaction as long as slow infusion over 30min (SQ route is variably efficacious). Smaller doses (5mg) can be given if INR is 1.5–1.9 range. Doses 5mg and greater can cause relative warfarin resistance up to one week

v. In patients taking rivaroxaban and apixaban (direct thrombin inhibitors) with ICH, there is no known antidote for drug reversal

vi. Some centers use recombinant factor VIIa (rFVIIa) 15–90mcg/kg IVPB for rapid warfarin reversal in place of FFP or PCC, which rapidly normalizes INR but has a delayed rebound effect at 24hrs—making vitamin K administration important since hepatic synthesis of factors II, VII, IX, and X should be on the rise

c. Blood pressure management

i. For ICH, usually < 140–180 systolic acutely

ii. May be complicated by elevated ICP

iii. Use short acting agents such as nicardipine and labetalol, especially early after the bleed

8. Anticonvulsants if seizure (typically phenytoin) occurs but not as prophylactic outside of trauma

When to Consider Consulting a Neurologist

1. For any of these disorders
2. Unclear etiology of hemorrhage
3. Suspect nonconvulsive seizures or need for EEG
4. Neurological prognosis considerations

Care Transitions

1. If seizure occurred during ICH, review driving/reporting issues specific to your state
2. Neurologist referral for seizure diagnosis, continuation of anticonvulsant, and/or neurological deficits
3. Acute rehabilitation placement if patient is suitable
4. Consider subacute neuropsychology evaluation as deficits may be subtle

Other Considerations

1. Patients who have "hypertensive ICH" are at risk for future ICH, especially if blood pressure remains uncontrolled as an outpatient
2. Perioperative care
   a. NPO and withhold enteral feeding after midnight before surgery
   b. Hold antithrombotics if possible before neurosurgical procedures in general
   c. Continue home medications if possible, except antithrombotics and in some cases antiypertensives
   d. Seizure prophylaxis is determined by the treating neurosurgeon

Proposed Quality Metrics

1. Aspiration pneumonia precautions
   a. Npo until swallow evaluation
2. Ventilator associated pneumonia (VAP) "bundle"
   a. Raise head of bed to 30 degrees to prevent aspiration while intubated
   b. daily sedation vacation
   c. oral decontamination/cleaning
3. DVT/PE prevention treatment
   a. Initial and continued sequential (pneumatic) compression devices (SCD)
   b. Chemical thromboprophylaxis or heparinoids can be considered if there is no vascular source of bleeding (typically not for at least first 48 hours and only with neurosurgical agreement), or if bleeding source was fixed (aneurysm completely coiled and secured)

    c. Some neurosurgeons prefer to hold heparinoids in patients with freshly placed (i.e., 48 hours or less) indwelling brain catheters (ventricular catheters or ICP monitors) or after craniotomy (SAH clipping or SDH/EDH) until they are comfortable that the risk of ICH after surgery is minimal.

       i. Subcutaneous heparin 5000 units q12hrs to q8hrs is usually considered for chemical DVT prevention if discussed with the surgeon on postoperative day #1 or 2 and varies based on surgeon's preference

      ii. IVC filters can be placed in ICH patients with DVT who cannot receive full anticoagulation (IV heparin or warfarin INR 2.0-3.0)

   d. Pulmonary embolism (PE) in ICH patients despite SCDs should be evaluated based on the severity of PE.

       i. Non-acutely life-threating situation (e.g., mild hypoxemia but able to be supplemented with O_2) and hemodynamically unstable, discussion with the neurosurgeon about safety of starting IV heparin (no bolus, target aPTT 50–70 range initially) with a gradual transition to warfarin could be considered if there is cranial CT stability

      ii. Unstable massive PE

        1. ICH is a contraindication for intravenous TPA

        2. Other means

          a. IV heparin

          b. Endovascular radiological techniques of low dose intra-arterial TPA (20mg or less) or mechanical thrombectomy, followed by IVC filter placement

4. Stress-ulcer prophylaxis if patients receiving corticosteroids, history of peptic ulcer disease or individualized to each ICH patient (Cushing's ulcer)

5. Rehabilitation consultation for physical therapy

6. Appropriate counseling prior to percutaneous gastrostomy placement

7. Secondary prevention measures (e.g., antihypertensives)

7

Venous Sinus Thrombosis

Questions to Ask

1. When do I look for venous sinus thrombosis?
   a. A difficult diagnosis to make clinically
   b. Headache is common
   c. May present with focal neurological signs
   d. Seizure may be present
   e. Cranial nerve palsy (e.g. VI)
2. What are risk factors for venous sinus thrombosis?
   a. Hypercoagulable state
   b. Late pregnancy
   c. Early postpartum
   d. Dehydration
   e. After trauma
   f. Oral contraceptive use
   g. Post-lumbar puncture

Exam Findings

1. Seizure
2. Forgetfulness/nonspecific slowness
3. Focal neurologic deficit such as cranial nerve VI paresis

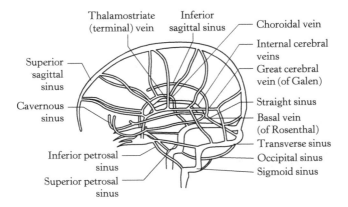

FIGURE 7.1

Venous Sinus Anatomy

Diagnostic Tests

1. Imaging (Figure 7.1)
   a. CT
      i. Noncontrast
         1. May show a venous stroke pattern
         2. Venous sinus clot may be difficult to notice {delta sign}
         3. May show hemorrhagic infarct (in venous pattern)
      ii. CT venogram
         1. Able to show the extent of clot well
   b. MRI
      i. Sensitive to venous pattern ischemia/infarction
      ii. Contrast
         1. May show enhancement of falx cerebri/tentorium
         2. MR venogram sensitive to presence of thrombus
2. Labs
   a. Depending on risk factors, hypercoagulable workup appropriate

Treatment Options

1. Little data
2. Anticoagulation
   a. Heparin typically used
   b. Transition to warfarin (depending on etiology)
   c. Newer anticoagulants not studied
3. Endovascular approaches rarely used
   d. Thrombolysis
   e. Mechanical clot disruption
   f. May be preferable if contraindications to anticoagulation

When to Consider Consulting a Neurologist

1. Appropriate to consult in most cases

Care Transitions

1. Follow-up for careful anticoagulation management
2. Anticonvulsant management if seizures occurred
3. Follow-up for determining time course of anticoagulation

Proposed Quality Metrics

1. Appropriate use of imaging in headache

8

Elevated Intracranial Pressure

Questions to Ask

1. What is normal and abnormal intracranial pressure (ICP)?
   a. Normal ICP: 0–20mmHg
   b. Abnormal ICP: >20mmHg
2. What are the signs of elevated intracranial pressure (ICP)?
   a. Clinical
      i. headache
      ii. nausea
      iii. sixth nerve palsy
      iv. depressed level of consciousness
      v. papilledema
      vi. increasing ICP and herniation
         1. coma
         2. unreactive and dilated pupil(s)
         3. posturing and then no motor response
   b. Imaging: CT findings typically include cerebral edema, flattening of the gyri or sulci, or a herniation syndrome (Figure 8.1)
      i. Uncal herniation
         1. uncus of the temporal lobe herniates over the tentorium cerebelli
         2. ipsilateral pupil dilatation and contralateral hemiparesis
         3. Pupillary findings can be contralateral if herniation of the uncus shifts the brainstem

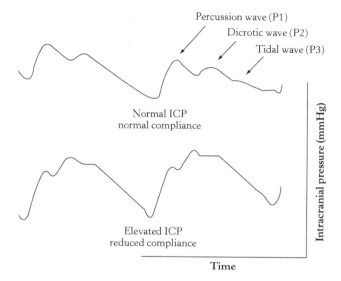

FIGURE 8.1

ICP waveforms, normal (top) and abnormal compliance (bottom).

Modified from O'Neal B Expert reviews.

    ii. Subfalcine
        1. brain tissue herniates laterally under the falx cerebri
        2. frontal lobe dysfunction and leg weakness
    iii. Diencephalic
        1. supratentorial diencephalon herniates into the posterior fossa, typically from global brain edema
        2. coma with varying degrees of pupillary dilatation depending on time course of the herniation
    iv. Foramen magnum
        1. coma with ataxic or apneic breathing
        2. tetraplegia from posterior fossa lesions
  c. ICP monitoring indications:
    i. severe traumatic brain injury (GCS 8 or less)
    ii. symptomatic hydrocephalus (e.g., from intracerebral hemorrhage with intraventricular hemorrhage)

3. Is there a role for surgical evacuation or ICP monitor placement?

a. Structural

i. surgical decompression of intracranial contents can immediately reduce ICP and improve intracranial compliance

ii. traumatic brain injury (TBI)—patients who present with TBI and persistent GCS 8 or less may benefit from ICP monitoring and management to keep ICP < 20mmHg and guide CPP

iii. subarachnoid hemorrhage from a ruptured brain aneurysm, AVM, or other vascular anomaly, with symptomatic hydrocephalus may benefit from an external ventricular drain (EVD) which also can monitor ICP

iv. hypertensive intraparenchymal bleeding typically does not require ICP monitoring, especially if located in the deep locations such as basal ganglia etc, unless there is concern about midline shift, mass effect, or hydrocephalus. If CSF obstructed or intraventricular extension, drainage is sometimes utilized

v. subdural hematoma (SDH) and epidural hematoma (EDH) may be spontaneous or traumatic in nature

1. if acutely symptomatic and/or >2cm maximal thickness with midline shift, these are often evacuated, with or without the need for ICP monitoring

vi. Decompressive hemicraniectomy

1. may be performed in patients 18–60 years of age

2. "malignant middle cerebral artery" infarction (>1/3 of MCA territory) or TBI with massive hemispheric edema, midline shift, herniation

3. can be a life-saving procedure in randomized, controlled trials but did not change stroke morbidity

Exam Findings

1. Physical examination/Assessment
   a. frequent neurologic monitoring (typically q1hr in the intensive care unit) provided by nursing staff that includes serial Glasgow Coma Scale (GCS) checks, and neurological examinations
   b. 2-point drop in the GCS sum scale which is not due to medications or other factors should raise suspicion for neurological deterioration or worsening ICP
   c. Monitor for development of new neurological lateralizing/localizing ("focal") findings on examination, especially cranial nerve findings such as dilation of one or both pupils or new hemiparesis
   d. Airway and global neurologic assessment such as Glasgow coma scale (GCS), patients with GCS 8 or less maybe considered for endotracheal intubation for airway protection to prevent aspiration pneumonia via rapid sequence intubation (RSI) protocol
2. Suspicion of trauma
   a. Battle's sign—ecchymosis behind mastoid
   b. raccoon eyes periorbital ecchymosis
   c. CSF leak from the ear or nose
   d. skull deformities
   e. cervical spine for step-off (palpable fracture) or instability
   f. chest, abdomen, and extremities should be examined for signs of trauma

Diagnostic Tests

1. Imaging
   a. noncontrast head CT is the most commonly used test to evaluate for worsening cerebral edema, infarction, or hemorrhage, mass effect with midline shift

b. the blood pattern of ICH typically predicts possible underlying pathologies

c. MRI with contrast if unknown cause of bleeding. In patients older than 70 years of age, gradient echo sequences can help reveal CAA pathology

2. Labs

a. serum osmolarity and electrolytes at baseline and frequently (q4-6hrs) if providing osmotherapy (mannitol or hypertonic saline)

b. serum creatinine at baseline and daily if performing osmotherapy to screen for renal failure

Treatment Algorithm

1. ABCs—airway, breathing, circulation

2. Head-neck position neutral, not in extreme lateral, flexion, or extension, with no constrictive ties around neck or jugular compression, and head of bed (HOB) >30 degrees to optimize jugular venous outflow and reduce ICP

3. CPP optimization

a. CPP = MAP –ICP

b. MAP—can be raised to offset ICP with pressors/vasoactive agents if needed

c. lower ICP

i. open CSF drain if present

ii. mannitol or hypertonic saline administration

4. Osmotherapy

a. frequent sodium monitoring and/or plasma osmolality

i. target sodium in patients who had prior normal serum sodium is 145–155

ii. If sodium is 155 or higher, typically osmotherapy is withheld or stopped and another means of controlling ICP is suggested

      iii. Patients often develop a hypernatremic hyperchloremic state after repeated doses of hypertonic saline

   b. Mannitol 20% solution 50grams to 100grams

      i. IVPB PRN signs of clinical herniation (extensor or flexor), enlargement and loss of reactivity of one pupil

      ii. may be repeated if clinical signs return q4–6hrs but need frequent sodium, electrolyte and osmolality checks

   c. Hypertonic saline boluses

      i. 14.6% 24ml or 48ml via central line if signs of herniation or elevated ICP sustained >20mmHg

      ii. 23.4% 15ml or 30ml via central line if signs of herniation or elevated ICP sustained >20mmHg

5. Surgical decompression of SDH, EDH are considered if symptomatic (and for some ICH patients such as those with cerebellar hemorrhage)

6. Placement of EVD for symptomatic hydrocephalus

7. Avoid secondary brain-insults

   a. hypoxemia (with mechanical ventilation if necessary)

   b. hypoglycemia

   c. hypotension (cerebral perfusion pressure [CPP] <60 mmHg)

8. Anticonvulsants if seizure (phenytoin) occurred at onset

When to Consider Consulting a Neurosurgeon or a Neurologist

1. Neurosurgeon or neurointensivist (if available): Patients who have suspected ICP elevation on clinical grounds and/or abnormal neuroimaging findings (CT with brain hemorrhage)

2. Neurosurgeon: A patient who is at risk for or acutely herniating with symptomatic mass lesion such as a ICH, SDH, EDH

3. Consultation with a neurologist is reasonable if a seizure occurred or if there are questions about management of antiepileptic medications (AED)

Care Transitions

1. Most patients with elevated ICP are admitted to the intensive care unit (ICU)
2. If a seizure occurs during the initial ICH or during hospitalization, review driving/reporting issues specific to your state before discharge home and other safety aspects of seizures
3. Consider consulting a neurologist for seizure diagnosis, or long-term continuation of anticonvulsant before discharge or in the outpatient followup setting
4. Consider rehabilitation placement following hospitalization

Other Considerations

1. Patients who have hypertensive ICH are at risk for recurrent ICH, especially if blood pressure remains uncontrolled
2. Perioperative care
   a. NPO and withhold enteral feeding after midnight before surgery
   b. Hold antithrombotics if possible before neurosurgical procedures
   c. Continue home medications if possible, except antithrombotics and antihypertensives
   d. Seizure prophylaxis is determined by the treating neurologist or neurosurgeon

Proposed Quality Metrics

1. Aspiration pneumonia precautions, avoidance of PO intake (pills or food) until formal swallow assessment is performed by nurse, speech pathologist or physician

2. Ventilator associated pneumonia (VAP) "bundle" in intubated patients
   a. Raise head of bed to 30 degrees to prevent gastric reflux aspiration while intubated
   b. daily sedation vacation
   c. oral decontamination/cleaning
3. DVT/PE prevention treatment
   a. initial and continued sequential (pneumatic) compression devices (SCD)
   b. Chemical thromboprophylaxis or heparinoids can be considered if there is no bleeding after ICP monitor placement or after craniotomy with neurosurgical agreement, or if bleeding source was fixed (aneurysm completely coiled and secured)
   c. Some neurosurgeons prefer to hold heparinoids in patients with freshly placed (i.e., 48hrs or less) indwelling brain catheters (ventricular catheters or ICP monitors) or after craniotomy (SAH clipping or SDH/EDH) until they are comfortable that the risk of ICH after surgery is minimal
      i. Subcutaneous heparin 5000units BID to q8hrs is usually considered for chemical DVT prevention if discussed with the surgeon on postoperative day #1 or 2 and varies based on surgeon's preference
      ii. IVC filters can be placed in ICH patients with DVT who cannot receive full anticoagulation (IV heparin or warfarin INR 2.0–3.0)
4. Stress-ulcer prophylaxis if patients receiving corticosteroids, history of peptic ulcer disease or individualized to each ICH patient (Cushing's ulcer)
5. Rehabilitation consultation for physical therapy, strengthening, gait training, assistive devices, bed mobility— if ICP is under control; physical or occupational therapy may

also be able to do passive range of motion of the shoulders and limbs to prevent contractures

6. Documentation of regular review of goals of care
7. Blood pressure goals short-term (i.e., within 2 weeks) and long-term in outpatient setting, and communicated to patient, care-giver, and the outpatient physician or team

9

CNS Demyelinating Disorders

Introduction

1. Multiple sclerosis (MS): A central nervous system demyelinating disorder affecting primarily the white matter of the brain and spinal cord as well as the optic nerves
   a. common in younger individuals with a female predominance
   b. most common form is Relapsing-Remitting MS: characterized by discrete attacks of neurologic dysfunction corresponding to acute areas of inflammation in the central nervous system
   c. secondary-progressive MS form often follows and is characterized by the absence of acute inflammation or discrete attacks
      i. progressive neurologic disability ensues with progressive atrophy seen on imaging
2. Neuromyelitis optica: A distinct demyelinating disorder with many overlapping clinical features with MS that affects mainly the spinal cord and optic nerves
   a. associated with an antibody directed against a water channel, aquaporin-4
3. Optic neuritis: An acute attack of demyelination of the optic nerve characterized by usually monocular visual loss and pain with eye movement

a. may herald the onset of other CNS demyelinating disorders (MS, neuromyelitis optica); may be part of other systemic diseases, or occur in isolation
4. Acute disseminated encephalomyelitis: A fulminant, monophasic attack of central nervous system demyelination which may be triggered in response to systemic infection or vaccination

Questions to Ask

1. History of previous attacks of focal neurologic dysfunction usually lasting days to weeks
   a. including bladder dysfunction, visual loss, weakness, imbalance, incoordination, or numbness
2. Family history of demyelinating disease, other autoimmune disorders, or unexplained neurologic conditions
3. Worsening of neurologic dysfunction with heat can occur in some patients with MS but is not a sensitive finding
4. Recent systemic infection or metabolic perturbation which could trigger a "pseudo flare" (see below)

Exam Findings

1. Evidence of focal findings localizing to the central nervous system
2. Optic neuritis
   a. poor visual acuity in one eye
   b. color desaturation, usually measured by presenting a red stimulus to the patient and comparing the color perceived in each eye
   c. afferent pupillary defect can be detected using the "swinging flashlight test"

i. When a light is moved from the unaffected to the affected eye, bilateral pupillary dilation will occur

Diagnostic Tests

1. Imaging
   a. MRI with contrast of the central nervous system is the preferred modality for diagnosis
      i. white matter lesions throughout the central nervous system are non-specific for MS, but suggestive sites of involvement include the corpus callosum, periatrial region, and spinal cord
         1. in MS, only around 1 in every 9 lesions will be symptomatic; therefore, many patients will present with numerous asymptomatic lesions at the time of first attack
      ii. the addition of contrast allows for visualization of acute areas of demyelination corresponding to new symptoms
      iii. some patients with MS will present with so-called "pseudo-flares" where old lesions will become symptomatic in the setting of systemic derangement (e.g. UTI)
         1. in these cases, no contrast-enhanced lesions will be seen and treatment is targeted to the underlying metabolic disorder
   b. MRI with contrast of the optic nerves can be useful in acute optic neuritis but is usually not necessary to make the diagnosis
   c. in acute disseminated encephalomyelitis, multiple enhancing lesions may be present on MRI including in the deep grey nuclei such as the thalamus
   d. if sarcoid is suspected, CT or MRI of the chest should be considered to look for characteristic hilar lymphadenopathy

2. Labs
   a. Used to exclude mimics in MS
      i. sarcoid: angiotensin converting enzyme (ACE)
      ii. Lyme disease: serum Lyme antibodies
      iii. syphilis: serum RPR
      iv. Other autoimmune disorders: Sjogren's antibodies, ANA
   b. serum aquaporin-4 antibodies in suspected neuromyelitis optica
3. Lumbar puncture
   a. useful to exclude other infectious etiologies
   b. typically demonstrates lymphocytic pleocytosis in MS (<50 cells)
      i. In ADEM, the pleocytosis may be more impressive (>100 cells)
   c. oligoclonal bands (OCBs) and IG index must be sent in tandem with corresponding serum samples
      i. abnormal results are not specific to MS, but provide supportive information in the right clinical setting
         1. early in the course of the illness, may be negative
4. Visual Evoked Potentials (VEPs)
   a. demonstrate physiologic evidence of previous attacks of (often unrecognized) optic neuritis
      i. provide additional supportive evidence of MS
   b. optical coherence tomography (OCT) is emerging as an even more sensitive test for the thinning of the optic nerve fiber layer that accompanies MS and neuromyelitis optica

Treatment Options

1. Multiple sclerosis and neuromyelitis optica
   a. for acute attacks resulting in severe neurologic dysfunction, intravenous corticosteroids are often used (e.g., 1 gram of methylprednisolone daily for 3–5 days)

    i. evidence suggests this treatment has no substantial effect on long-term outcome or recovery from acute attacks; it likely merely shortens the duration of the attack

        1. therefore, it should only be used when attacks are disabling

        2. some clinicians use oral regimens which are less studied

  b. when attacks are refractory to corticosteroids, plasmapheresis or intravenous immunoglobulin (IVIg) are often considered

  c. chronic treatment includes disease-modifying treatments such as beta-interferons and glatiramir acetate, although various effective immunomodulatory drugs are often employed

    i. becoming more common to initiate treatment even after a single clinical attack as field moves toward aggressive early therapy to prevent disability

2. Acute disseminated encephalomyelitis

  a. treatment typically begins with intravenous corticosteroids with consideration of plasmapheresis or intravenous immunoglobulin

3. Optic neuritis

  a. Attacks are treated with intravenous methylprednisolone (1 gram for 3 days) followed by an oral steroid taper per the results of the optic neuritis treatment trial

When to Consider Consulting a Neurologist

1. When faced with an acute attack which is severe or refractory to initial treatment
2. Acute disseminated encephalomyelitis
3. Suspected MS mimic or uncertainty as to the diagnosis

Care Transitions

1. All patients with a first attack of demyelination should follow up with a neurologist for discussion of potential initiation of disease-modifying therapies; many times this discussion can occur in an outpatient setting
2. Screen for bladder dysfunction with post-void residual, especially in the setting of spinal cord disease
3. Physical and occupational therapy referrals
4. For those with new visual loss, consideration of safe driving is important

Proposed Quality Metrics

1. Patients with an acute attack of optic neuritis should be treated with intravenous corticosteroids
2. Patients with suspected first attack of demyelination should undergo MRI of the brain and/or spine (depending on symptoms) with contrast
3. Patients presenting with disabling acute attacks of demyelination should be treated with corticosteroids

Meningitis and Encephalitis

Questions to Ask

1. What is the difference between meningitis and encephalitis?
   a. Meningitis is an infection of the meninges, spaces, and tissues external to the brain
   b. Encephalitis is an infection of the brain itself.
2. Is a CT (or other imaging) necessary before a lumbar puncture?
   a. Those at risk for abnormal findings on imaging include
      i. adults age >60
      ii. abnormal level of consciousness
      iii. immunocompromised state
      iv. history of a CNS lesion
      v. seizure within one week
      vi. focal signs on neurological examination
3. How do you correct CSF protein for blood?
   a. subtract 0.01 g from the protein for every 1000 RBC's
   b. ideally, the red blood cell count will decrease in sequential tubes

Exam Findings

1. Headache
2. Meningismus—irritation of the meninges causes neck stiffness/pain on range of motion

3. Kernig's sign—flexing the hip at 90 degrees, then extending the knee causes neck pain
4. Brudzinski's sign—neck flexion causes the patient to flex at the hips and knees
5. Photophobia—light causes pain
6. Phonophobia—sounds cause pain
7. Nonspecific signs of infection—fever, etc

Diagnostic Tests

1. Imaging
   a. see *Questions to Ask* section for indications for imaging
   b. rule out potential cause for herniation with lumbar puncture
   c. rule out abscess or mass lesion
   d. rule out hemorrhage (may indicate herpes encephalitis with temporal lobe predilection)
   e. MRI more sensitive than CT for parenchymal abnormality
2. Lumbar puncture
   a. a necessity for definite diagnosis of meningitis
   b. may not diagnose encephalitis, but is typically abnormal
   c. opening pressure when high provides useful information that guides management
3. Labs
   a. blood
      i. CBC to evaluate white count/differential
      ii. CMP
   a. Cerebrospinal fluid (Table 10.1)
      i. cell count and differential (neutrophils more common with bacterial infection, monoctyes/lymphocytes more common with viral/fungal)
      ii. protein—nonspecific but typically elevated in infection

TABLE 10.1 Cerebrospinal fluid findings in meningitis

Meningitis	Pressure (mmH$_2$O)	Leucocytes/µl	Protein (g/l)	Glucose (mmol/l)
Acute bacterial	Usually elevated	Several hundred to more than 60 00; usually a few thousand but occasionally <100 (especially meningococcal or early in disease). Polymorphonuclears predominate.	Usually 1 to 5, occasionally more than 10	0.2 to 2.2 in most cases (in the absence of hyperglycaemia)
Tubercilous	Usually elevated; may be low with dynamic block in advanced stages	0 to 800; average 50. Lymphocytes predominate	Nearly always elevated usually 1 to 2; may be much higher if dynamic block	Usually reduced; < 2.5 in three-Quarters of cases
Cryptococcal	Usually elevated	5 to a few hundred; but may be more than 1000, particularly with lymphocytic choriomeningitis. Lymphocytes predominate but there may be more than 80 per cent polymorphonuclears in the first few days	Usally 0.2 to 5; averge 1	Reduced in most cases; average 1.7 (in absence of hyperglycaemia)
Viral	Normal to moderately	Averege 500. Usually lymphocytes; rarely polymorphonuclear	Frequently normal or slightly elevated; < 1; may show greater elevation in severe cases	Normal (reduced in one-quarters of cases of mumps and herpes simplex)

TABLE 10.1 (Continued)

Meningitis	Pressure (mmH$_2$O)	Leucocytes/µl	Protein (g/l)	Glucose (mmol/l)
Syphilitic (acute)	Usally elevated	Average 500. Usually lympho-cytes; rarely polymoerphonuclear	Average 1	Normal (rarely reduced)
Cysticercosis	Often increased; low	Increased mononuclears and poly-morphonuclears with 2 to 7 per cent eosinophilia in about half of cases	Usually 0.5 to 2	Reduced in half of cases
Sarcoid	Normal to consid-erably elevated	0 to fewer than 100 mononuclear cells	Slight to moderate elevation	Reduced in half of cases
Tumor	Normal or elevated	0 to several hundred mononucle-ars plus malignant cells	Elevated often to high levels	Normal or greatly reduced (low in three-quarters of carcinomatous

Cerebrospinal fluid immunoglobulins are commonly increased in all of the above (including carcinomatous meningitis) as well as in multiple sclerosis and central nervous system vasculitis.

Cerebrospinal fluid immunoglobulins are assessed by the IgG index: (IgG (cerebrospinal fluid)×albumin (serum))/(IgG serum×albumin(cerebrospinal fluid)). The normal index is <0.65.

Oligocional bands (with gel electrophoresis) present in cerebrospinal fluid but absent in serum are also a measure of abnormally increased cerebrospinal fluid immunoglobulins synthesized within the CNS).

     iii. glucose—usually normal in viral, low in bacterial and fungal or mycobacterial

     iv. gram stain—may help identify organism

     v. cultures—both bacterial and viral

     vi. cryptococcal antigen—in the immunosuppressed

     vii.coccidioides (serum and CSF antibodies), histoplasma (urinary antigen)—in endemic locations +/- immunosuppression

     viii. tuberculosis—culture/visualization

     ix. syphilis

       1. VDRL specific>sensitive

       2. FTA-ABS sensitive>specific

     x. viral studies (PCR)

       3. HSV

       4. enterovirus

       5. Epstein-Barr virus

       6. CMV

       7. HIV

     xi. many other possible etiologies/tests

4. EEG

   a. consider with altered mental status or even subtle personality/ cognitive changes

Treatment Options

1. Do not let testing (imaging or lumbar puncture) delay therapy
2. Antibiotics
   a. be aware of what organisms are most common in your community
   b. empiric therapy
     i. vancomycin + ceftriaxone or cefotaxime + ampicillin (to cover listeria, important in older patients and those who are pregnant)

      ii. vancomycin + ceftazidime (in post op neurosurgery patients)

      iii. vancomycin + ceftazidime + ampicillin (in immuo-compromised)

3. Steroids

    i. give before or with first dose of antibiotics

    ii. helpful in pneumococcal, tuberculous meningitis in adults and H. flu in children

    iii. dexamethasone 10mg q6 hours x 4 days or until culture negative for the above organisms

4. Antivirals

    i. with a compatible CSF and clinical presentation

    ii. most viral meningitis is benign and self-limited

    iii. acyclovir IV 10mg/kg q8hrs for HSV

    iv. ganciclovir IV 5mg/kg q12hrs for CMV

5. Anticonvulsants

    a. none empirically

When to Consider Consulting a Neurologist

1. uncertain diagnosis
2. unusual features to the infection
3. decreased level of consciousness
4. focal neurological findings

Care Transitions

1. Neurology follow up if consulted in the hospital, especially if seizures occurred

Other Considerations

1. Select non-infectious etiologies of meningitis
    a. malignancies

    b. medications
        i. NSAIDs
        ii. IVIG
        iii. trimethoprim/sulfamethoxazole
        iv. ciprofloxacin
    c. rheumatologic
        i. lupus
        ii. Behçet's
        iii. Sjögrens
        iv. primary CNS angiitis
        v. sarcoidosis
    d. postoperative neurosurgery
2. recurrent meningitis
    a. Mollaret's due to recurrent HSV-2
3. Select other causes of encephalitis
    a. flaviviruses (mosquito-borne)
        i. West Nile
        ii. St. Louis
        iii. Japanese
    b. Epstein-Barr
    c. Rocky Mountain spotted fever
    d. progressive multifocal leukoencephalopathy
        i. due to JC virus
        ii. associated with immunosuppressants
4. Select non-infectious encephalitis
    a. Limbic encephalitis
        i. usually due to malignancy or autoimmunity
        ii. "limbic" symptoms such as memory loss, personality change
        iii. seizures common
    b. steroid-responsive encephalopathy (previously called Hashimoto's)
5. Patients at risk for subsequent complications
    a. hydrocephalus

b. venous stroke

c. seizure

d. hearing loss

e. focal neurological deficits

Proposed Quality Metrics

1. Timeliness and appropriate selection of antibiotics
2. Timeliness, appropriateness, and duration of steroid use
3. Appropriate use of imaging

11

Spinal Epidural Abscess

Questions to Ask

1. Is there evidence of neurological compromise?
   a. a careful, detailed exam is critically important
   b. if abnormalities are found, represents a potential surgical emergency
   c. history
      i. lancinating/shooting pain
      ii. bowel or bladder dysfunction
2. Does the patient have an identifiable risk factor?
   a. epidural catheters/injections are a significant risk factor
   b. spine surgery
   c. cellulitis/soft tissue infections
   d. IV drug abuse
   e. bacteremia
   f. immunocompromised state

Exam Findings

1. Back pain
   a. common with spinal epidural abscess
   b. a very uncommon cause of back pain
2. Fever
   a. may be absent
   b. should raise a red flag when present in patients with back pain

3. Neurological exam
    a. abnormalities should prompt imaging and further evaluation
    b. may have a sensory level useful to check soft touch or pin prick, vibration sense throughout spinal levels (cervical, thoracic, lumbar and sacral)
    c. motor deficits
        i. important to test for
        ii. may be difficult in setting of significant pain
    d. reflex asymmetry
        i. may help define the level involved

Diagnostic Tests

1. Imaging
    1. MRI is most sensitive, and contrast unnecessary (Figure 11.1)
        a. CT an alternative, intravenous contrast needed
        b. plain X rays typically not helpful, but may show bony disease (osteomyelitis)
2. Lumbar puncture
    a. low yield and potential to introduce infection into intradural space
3. Labs
    a. blood
        i. CBC to evaluate white count/differential
        ii. ESR typically elevated
        iii. C reactive protein usually elevated
        iv. cultures to identify bacteremia/causative organism

Treatment Options

1. Antibiotics
    a. S. aureus is the most common organism

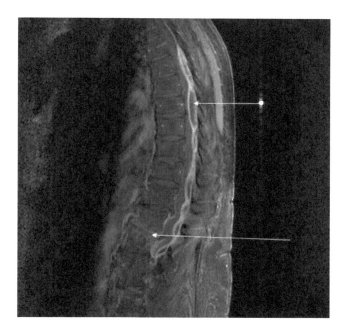

FIGURE 11.1

T1-Gd enhanced MRI of epidural abscess in mid dorsal spine compressing the spinal cord (top arrow). Loss of disc space and bone change at site of discitis (bottom arrow).

    b. tailor therapy once an organism identified
    c. empiric therapy
       i. vancomycin + ceftriaxone or cefotaxime or ceftazidime + metronidazole
       ii. empiric coverage (as above) for MRSA is typically appropriate
2. Drainage
    a. surgery
       i. emergent surgical consultation needed with evidence of neurological compromise as deficits may become permanent

    b. interventional radiology
       i. typically CT guided approach
      ii. aspirate for culture, drainage

When to Consider Consulting a Neurologist

1. Uncertain diagnosis
2. Unusual features to the infection
3. Focal or unclear neurological findings

Care Transitions

1. Transfer to a center with surgical/interventional support if evidence of neurological compromise
2. Many patients will see an improvement in their deficits over time, therefore transition to an inpatient rehabilitation/ neurorehabilitation facility is encouraged

Other Considerations

Proposed Quality Metrics

1. Timeliness and appropriate selection of antibiotics
2. Timeliness of surgical evaluation
3. Appropriate discharge location

12

Seizure

Questions to Ask

1. What kind of seizure was it?
   a. focal—affecting a portion of the brain and not affecting level of consciousness
   b. complex focal with dyscognitive features—affecting a portion of the brain and does affect level of consciousness
   c. generalized—affecting both hemispheres of the brain, leading to a decreased level of consciousness
2. Is there a prior history of seizure?
   a. epilepsy
   b. drug/alcohol use/withdrawal
3. Is the seizure due to a discernible cause?
   a. structural
      i. acute/chronic stroke
      ii. acute/chronic head injury
      iii. abscess, tumor, etc.
   b. electrolyte abnormality

Exam Findings

1. Evidence of seizure
   a. tongue lacerations
   b. other injuries

    c. post-ictal paralysis—that is, Todd's paralysis (may mimic a stroke)
2. Clues to other underlying conditions that may predispose to seizure
3. Medic-alert bracelet identifying patient as an epileptic

Diagnostic Tests

1. Imaging
   a. always perform for patients with unknown history or new onset seizures
   b. MRI preferred if it will not introduce a delay in care/evaluation
2. Labs
   a. electrolyte abnormality
      i. sodium
      ii. calcium
      iii. magnesium
   b. serum glucose (always assure that this has been done as hypoglycemia commonly leads to seizures)
   c. toxicology screening
   d. anti-epileptic drug levels—in patients with epilepsy
   e. lumbar puncture
      i. Consider in immunocompromised, infection of uncertain cause, persistent abnormal mental status
3. EEG
   a. not typically useful for provoked seizures (result of an acute process)
   b. not typically useful for known epileptics who have returned to baseline mental status
   c. useful for patients who have had a seizure with persistently abnormal mental status to exclude ongoing subclinical seizures
   d. somewhat helpful to predict seizure recurrence

Treatment Options

1. For a provoked seizure, treat the underlying provoking factor
2. For a first time non-provoked seizure, a medication may not be necessary
3. Choice of medication is a complex decision given drug interactions and side effect profiles
4. Acute medication choice may be temporary, and changed over time in the outpatient realm

When to Consider Consulting a Neurologist

1. Status epilepticus
2. Unclear seizure etiology

Care Transitions

1. Assure education about safety issues at discharge
2. Review driving/reporting issues specific to your state
3. Neurologist follow-up when no reversible cause of seizure found

Other Considerations

1. Risk of recurrence for unprovoked seizure
   a. 36–47% of patients will have another within 2 years (Berg, 1991)
2. Perioperative care
   a. continue medications as possible
   b. for prolonged NPO periods without an IV equivalent, consider short-term substitution with another medication

(benzodiazepines, fosphenytoin, valproic acid, lacosamide, levetiracetam)

Proposed Quality Metrics

1. Time to resolution of seizure and administration of anticonvulsants
2. Documentation of discussions of safety at discharge

13

Status Epilepticus

Questions to Ask

1. Is this status epilepticus?
   a. varying definitions, but essentially seizures that beget further seizures if not interrupted
   b. many use a definition of seizures lasting for more than 5 minutes
   c. formally defined by the International League against Epilepsy as 2 or more seizures during 30 minutes without full recovery
2. Why is it important to treat status epilepticus emergently?
   a. the longer seizures persist, the more difficult to treat they become
   b. convulsive status epilepticus
      i. brain damage
      ii. increased morbidity and mortality
   c. nonconvulsive status epilepticus
      i. data less clear, but poorer outcomes overall

Exam Findings

1. Typically seizures are obvious; however, may become very difficult to clinically recognize
2. Nonconvulsive status epilepticus may only manifest as altered mental status

Diagnostic Tests

1. Imaging
   a. MRI may show evidence of focal abnormality in area of seizure focus
2. Labs
   a. as in seizure section
3. EEG
   a. imperative for status epilepticus
   b. perform even if patient back to baseline, especially if no prior history of seizure
   c. patients without clear return to baseline may need serial EEGs or continuous EEG monitoring

Treatment Options

1. ABCs: Airway, Breathing, Circulation
2. Many anticonvulsants are respiratory suppressants, so need a low threshold for intubation
3. Assure appropriate intravenous access
4. See treatment algorithm (Figure 13.1)
   a. first line is lorazepam
   b. consider concomitant load of fosphenytoin
      i. Not 1 gram – use 18–20 mg/kg
   c. as seizures continue, there are multiple other drug options per the algorithm
   d. seizures may become clinically inapparent and EEG evaluation becomes necessary and may prompt transfer if subtle abnormalities are noted and the patient requires third line medications

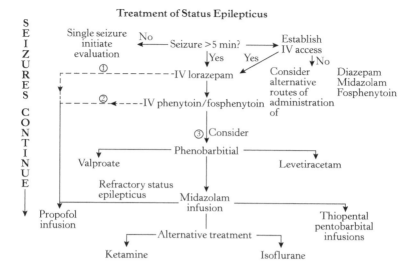

FIGURE 13.1

Algorithm for the treatment of status epilepticus. Treatment can proceed along several different pathways to obtain the most immediate seizure control.

When to Consider Consulting a Neurologist

1. All cases of status epilepticus

Care Transitions

1. Assure education about safety issues at discharge
2. Review driving/reporting issues specific to your state
3. Neurologist follow-up to help determine appropriate outpatient anticonvulsant regimen

Other Considerations

Proposed Quality Metrics

1. Time to resolution of seizure and administration of anticonvulsants
2. Appropriate use of EEG
3. Appropriate admitting unit (ability to closely monitor and manage airway if necessary—typically critical care)
4. Documentation of discussions of safety at discharge

Syncope

Questions to Ask

1. Ask the patient to describe the episode in detail
   a. What were you doing at the time? Were there triggering factors?
      i. Knowledge of the patient's activity can help identify possible causes of the syncopal episode
      ii. For example, if the patient was a young athletic male who had a syncopal episode while exercising, consider hypertrophic cardiomyopathy
   b. Was it vasovagal syncope?
      i. vasovagal syncope and some arrhythmias may leave time to lay down and avoid injury
      ii. other associated symptoms
         1. Did you feel cold and clammy?
         2. Did you have tunnel vision?
         3. Did you feel lightheaded?
   c. Did you feel any palpitations?
      i. may indicate an atrial dysrhythmia (i.e., atrial fibrillation with a rapid ventricular response) that decreased cardiac output and caused syncope
      ii. lack of palpitations with a sudden syncopal episode with no prodromal symptoms should make one think of potential ventricular dysrhythmias
   d. Did the episode occur with exertion?

        i. potential outflow tract obstruction (aortic stenosis, hypertrophic cardiomyopathy) or ventricular dysrhythmia

   e. How long did the episode last?

        i. In general, longer episodes associated with seizures.

        ii. Brief episodes are often linked to syncope due to atrial or ventricular dysrhythmias

   f. Did anyone witness the episode?

        i. invaluable information providing the exact circumstances of the syncopal episode

2. Have you ever had any similar episodes?

   a. may help differentiate malingering/conversion

   b. if stereotypic, may imply seizure

3. Was there postsyncopal confusion?

   a. may represent a post-ictal state from seizure

4. Is this patient high risk?

   a. risk stratification studies

        i. best known is the San Francisco Syncope Rule

          1. history of congestive heart failure

          2. hematocrit < 30%

          3. ECG abnormality

          4. history of dyspnea

          5. systolic blood pressure < 90mmHg at admission

        ii. The Osservatorio Epidemiologico sulla Sincope nel Lazio (OESIL) identified risk factors for death at one year

          1. abnormal ECG

          2. history of cardiovascular disease

          3. age > 65 years old

          4. no prodromal symptoms

        iii. Risk stratification of Syncope in the Emergency department (ROSE) utilizes the acronym BRACES

          1. BNP ≥ 300pg/mL

          2. Bradycardia ≤ 50/minute (prehospital or emergency department)

3. rectal examination with evidence of fecal occult blood (FOB)
4. anemia (hemoglobin ≤ 9g/dL)
5. chest pain in association with the syncopal episode
6. ECG with a Q wave (except in lead III)
7. oxygen saturation ≤ 94% on room air

Exam Findings

1. General appearance
   a. unexplained bruising or trauma
      i. lends credence to the episode
   b. tongue lacerations
      i. may imply seizure (along with incontinence)
      ii. presence or absence does not rule out or confirm seizure
2. Orthostasis
3. Cardiac murmurs or extra sounds
4. Cardiac rhythm
5. Mental status assessment
   a. evidence of confusion or disorientation
6. Focal neurologic deficits

Diagnostic Tests

1. The following should be done in every patient presenting with syncope:
   a. accu-check
   b. ECG
   c. orthostatic blood pressure
2. Labs
   a. Hemoglobin can be obtained as severe anemia can cause orthostatic hypotension, leading to syncope

b. There has been some investigation into the role of brain natriuretic peptide (BNP) in the evaluation of syncope

    i. One study demonstrated that elevated BNP levels correlate with increased cardiovascular risk and all-cause mortality

3. Imaging

a. other diagnostic tests (echocardiogram, CT, carotid Duplex, MRI, tilt table testing) only based on the patient's history and physical examination findings

    i. data supports directed diagnostic testing for syncope

    ii. a "shotgun" approach of ordering multiple diagnostic tests does not increase the diagnostic yield, only adding cost

4. Other

a. Those patients in whom cardiac dysrhythmias are suspected (but not documented on telemetry) should be evaluated by cardiology and set up with outpatient cardiac monitoring. Patients with a prodrome suggestive of dysrhythmia, syncope with exertion, ECG changes, or a history of structural heart disease should be further evaluated

Treatment Options

1. Treatment options will depend upon the likely underlying etiology

a. vasovagal syncope

    i. counseling to avoid potential triggers as much as possible

b. orthostasis

    i. counseling regarding postural changes

    ii. avoid diuretics and medications that can potentially cause orthostasis

    iii. consider fludrocortisone and/or midodrine

        1. follow for development of supine hypertension
        2. follow electrolytes
   c. structural heart disease (i.e., aortic stenosis)
      i. determine the severity of the disease and timing of potential surgical or other intervention
   d. dysrhythmias (particularly bradydysrhythmia)
      i. evaluate for pacemaker placement or medication to control tachydysrhythmias

When to Consider Consulting a Neurologist

1. Focal neurologic deficit
2. Evidence or suspicion of seizure

Care Transitions

1. Most patients with syncope will be able to return home
2. Those patients who require further evaluation (i.e., those with potential cardiac dysrhythmias) will need clear follow-up, involving both the involved subspecialist (cardiologist, neurologist) and the patient's primary care physician

Other Considerations

1. Accurate diagnosis of a syncopal episode is important
2. An appropriate history and physical, with basic laboratory testing, can establish a probable etiology of the syncope in around 70% of cases
3. Many patients (15–40%, depending upon the series) will have no discernible cause for their syncope

Proposed Quality Metrics

1. A review of history and physical to evaluate adequacy of data gathering and physical examination in patients presenting with syncope
2. Routine risk stratification of syncopal patients
3. Length of stay
4. Evidence of recurrent syncope
5. Appropriate use of diagnostic modalities (lab and imaging)

Headache

Questions to Ask

1. Was the onset sudden or gradual?
   a. Sudden headaches, such as the classic "thunderclap" headache, may heighten the suspicion of subarachnoid hemorrhage
2. Was the headache preceded by any aura or prodromal symptoms?
   a. consistent with migraine headache
3. Has the patient suffered from headaches in the past?
4. Does the pain get worse with exertion?
   a. this, along with pain that is "band-like" or a "heaviness" in the head and shoulder—think of tension headache
   b. sudden onset during exertion worrisome for bleeding
5. Where is the pain located?
   a. classic headache locations
      i.   unilateral = migraine
      ii. bilateral = tension
      iii. temporal = temporal arteritis
      iv. orbital or supraorbital and unilateral = cluster
      v.   neck and shoulders = tension
      vi. meningismus = subarachnoid hemorrhage or infection
6. How does the patient describe the pain?
   a. throbbing = migraine
   b. muscle tenderness = tension

    c. associated with a pulsatile noise = dissection

7. Are there any associated signs and symptoms accompanying the headache?
   a. visual changes
   b. nausea with or without emesis
   c. photophobia
   d. sonophobia
   e. lacrimation
   f. rhinorrhea
8. Are there any triggers for the headache?
   a. activity
   b. food
   c. alcohol
9. Has the patient had recent trauma?
   a. raises concern for arterial dissection.
10. Are there any changes in sleep or exercise?
    a. may be a trigger for migraine
11. Have the headaches changed at all in character from prior headaches?
    a. should change the patient's evaluation, as a different type of headache may be affecting the patient
12. Does the patient have any active infections or has the patient recently been treated for an active infection?
13. Does the patient have a history of HIV?
    a. raises suspicion of infection, possibly leading to elevated intracranial pressure
14. Findings that may indicate a serious underlying problem:
    a. a headache that occurs suddenly and reaches maximal intensity quickly
    b. a patient describing the headache as the "worst in my life"
    c. a patient without similar severe headaches in the past
    d. presence of focal neurologic findings
    e. presence of fever
    f. mental status changes

g. history of coagulopathy—venous sinus thrombosis

h. history of jaw claudication or blurred/darkened vision—temporal arteritis

Exam Findings

1. Pay attention to the patient's general appearance
   a. a patient lying still in a quiet and dark room may indicate a migraine headache (photophobia and phonophobia)
   b. a toxic-appearing patient may have meningitis
   c. Is there any evidence of trauma?
   d. Does the patient have obvious focal neurologic deficits?
2. General examination findings
   a. Assess mental status, evaluating for changes in mental status or personality
   b. Does the patient have any muscle tenderness?
   c. Is there any tenderness on palpation of the scalp indicating tension headache?
   d. Is there tenderness around the temporal arteries indicating temporal arteritis?
   e. Neck stiffness and meningismus suggest meningitis.
3. A good eye examination is important, evaluating for evidence of papilledema (blurring of the optic disks)
   a. presence of papilledema indicates elevated intracranial pressure due to mass lesion, CNS infection, or pseudotumor cerebri
4. Is there any evidence of a seizure?
   a. tongue laceration
   b. sore muscles
   c. other injuries?
5. A full neurologic examination should be performed, evaluating the patient for subtle defects that may indicate underlying mass lesion

6. Examination findings that may indicate a serious underlying problem:
   a. focal neurologic deficits
   b. papilledema
   c. meningismus
   d. toxic or ill-appearing patient
   e. altered consciousness or personality
   f. evidence of trauma

Diagnostic Tests

1. If the patient has any high-risk features based on history or examination, a CT or MRI should be performed to evaluate for the presence of mass lesion or underlying CNS abnormality.
   a. routine CNS imaging should not be performed in patients with a normal neurologic examination and no "red flags" on history
2. Indications for lumbar puncture
   a. suspicion of meningitis or CNS infection
   b. suspicion of subarachnoid hemorrhage with negative neuroimaging
   c. reminder that a CT scan is not necessary prior to the LP if there is no evidence of increased intracranial pressure (see imaging section)
3. CTA or MRA may be indicated if the patient has suspected arterial dissection or aneurysm
   a. patient may present with a history of recent (even very minor) trauma and a headache that occurs suddenly with exertion or exercise

Treatment Options

1. Patients with high risk findings on history or physical examination should be admitted for further evaluation

    a. if there is suspected CNS infection, begin prompt antibiotic therapy (see chapter 10)

    b. neurology and neurosurgical evaluation are indicated in patients with suspected CNS lesions or hemorrhage

2. Patients without high risk findings who do not have migraine headaches should receive non-steroidal anti-inflammatory medications

3. Patients with migraine headaches may receive:

    a. options

      i. non-steroidal anti-inflammatories. A broad range of anti-inflammatories may be used (aspirin, ibuprofen, and naproxen); while patients may receive relief with diclofenac, it is probably best used as a second-line agent

      ii. ergotamine medications

      iii. triptans. These are available in different preparations (injectable, oral, sublingual, and intranasal)

      iv. anti-emetics as needed

    b. a step-wise approach to treatment is typically warranted. Most of these approaches will begin with a combination of an NSAID and an anti-emetic (such as metoclopramide) and escalate to a triptan if the patient does not experience relief

4. Cluster headaches may be aborted with oxygen therapy

    a. A standard treatment regimen is to deliver 100% oxygen via a non-rebreather mask to the patient for 15 minutes

    b. If this is not successful in aborting the cluster, triptans and octreotide have demonstrated efficacy in the treatment of cluster headaches

When to Consider Consulting a Neurologist

1. High risk history or physical examination findings that point toward possible:

    a. subarachnoid (or other intracranial) hemorrhage

      b. cervical artery dissection

      c. CNS lesion

  2. Refractory migraine headache (status migrainosus)

  3. Unusual headache

Care Transitions

1. For most headache patients, care transitions are straightforward with outpatient follow-up with the patient's primary care physician
2. Patients with underlying CNS abnormality or infection may require outpatient rehabilitation (PT/OT/speech) depending upon the presence and extent of focal neurologic findings and/or deconditioning
3. Patients with refractory headache may benefit from follow up with a headache specialist

Other Considerations

Proposed Quality Metrics

1. Appropriate utilization of CNS imaging

Delirium

Introduction

1. Delirium/Encephalopathy
   a. waxing and waning confusion of acute onset
   b. patients may have a hyperactive or hypoactive presentation
2. Very common condition in the hospital, especially among elderly and ICU patients
3. Results in increased length of stay, morbidity, costs, and subsequent mortality
4. An indicator of potential underlying cognitive impairment
5. Hallucinations and delusions are common in hyperactive form
   a. Important to differentiate from dementia/depression (Figure 16.1)

Questions to Ask

1. Is there a history of similar episodes?
   a. patients may have paradoxical reactions to specific medications
   b. may help identify other precipitating factors
2. Is there a history of cognitive impairment?
   a. a good question to ask in assessing risk for delirium since this is a major risk factor

	Delirium	Dementia	Depression
Onset	Acute	Insidious[a]	Variable
Course	Fluctuating	Often progressive	Diurnal variation
Reversibility	Frequently[b]	Not usually	Usually but can be recurrent
Level of consciousness	Impaired	Unimpaired until late stages	Generally unimpaired
Attention/memory	Inattention is primary with poor memory	Poor memory without marked inattention except in end-stage illness	Mild attention problems, inconsistent pattern—depressive pseudodementia, memory intact with formal testing
Affect	Lability	No clear pattern	Flattening
Hallucinations	Usually visual; can be auditory, tactile, gustatory, olfactory	Can be visual or auditory	Usually auditory
Delusions	Fleeting, fragmented, and usually persecutory often relate to immediate environment or impending danger	Paranoid, often fixed, relate to misconceptions	Complex and mood congruent e.g. themes of guilt or nihilism

[a]Except for large strokes that can be abrupt and Lewy Body Dementia which can be subacute.
[b]Can be chronic (paraneoplastic syndrome, central nervous system adverse events of medications, severe brain damage).

FIGURE 16.1

Differential diagnosis of delirium vs other common neuropsychiatric conditions

3. Does the patient have other predisposing factors to developing delirium?
   a. advanced age
   b. problems with sensory perception—poor hearing, vision
   c. withdrawal risk—narcotics, alcohol
   d. surgery
   e. malnutrition at baseline
4. Do we have a complete medication list?
   a. critical to review both new medications as well as baseline medications
5. Is there evidence of an infection?
   a. delirium may be the only manifestation, especially in the elderly

Exam Findings

1. Mental status exam
   a. inattention is a hallmark of delirium
2. Careful neurological examination looking for any evidence of focality/asymmetry
3. General exam for evidence of trauma
   a. subdural hematoma may not present with an otherwise abnormal neurological exam
4. General exam for evidence of infection
5. General exam for evidence of withdrawal symptoms
6. Consider implementation of standardized screening
   a. Confusional Assessment Method (CAM)
   b. when used by nursing can help alert to incipient delirium

Diagnostic Tests

1. Labs
   a. CBC
      i. especially white count for a clue to infection or malignancy
   b. electrolytes
      i. multiple abnormalities may cause confusion, even when mildly abnormal in susceptible individuals
   c. creatinine
      i. renal failure may result in delirium
   d. hepatic enzymes
      i. may reveal occult liver disease
      ii. ammonia level may be useful
   e. TSH
      i. as an initial screen
   f. B12 levels
   g. cortisol
2. Imaging
   a. CT
      i. good screening exam, especially for intracranial or subdural hemmorhages
   b. MRI
      i. may be preferable in many cases if patient is cooperative
      ii. more sensitive for subtle abnormalities
3. Lumbar puncture
   a. useful to exclude infectious etiologies, most commonly encephalitis
4. EEG
   a. subclinical seizure increasingly recognized as a cause of delirium
   b. especially in the ICU

Treatment Options

1. Correct underlying cause if identified
2. Prevention/amelioration
   a. orientation clues
      i. clocks
      ii. calendars
      iii. Family members
   b. normalize sleep schedule as able
   c. avoid constipation
   d. avoid dehydration
   e. provide careful pain control
   f. minimize sedatives
   g. avoid restraints
   h. avoid bladder catheterization
3. Medications
   a. avoid if possible unless patient posing harm to themselves or staff
   b. similar efficacy between haloperidol and atypical antipsychotics
   c. care with cardiac patients, potential for precipitating arrhythmias
   d. many may increase mortality in the elderly and be evaluated for changes in follow-up
   e. benzodiazepines only for alcohol withdrawal

When to Consider Consulting a Neurologist

1. If concern for seizure or stroke
2. Difficult to control delirium
3. Unusual features of delirium
4. Underlying neurological disease that may worsen/precipitate delirium

Care Transitions

1. Assure close followup for re-evaluation of medication regimen
2. Evaluate for resolution of cognitive impairment
3. Consider subacute screening for underlying dementia or mild cognitive impairment

Proposed Quality Metrics

1. Fall rates
2. Length of stay for surgeries
3. Readmission rates for patients with delirium
4. Plan to discontinue antipsychotics if needed at the time of discharge
5. Formal care pathways in place to decrease development of delirium

17

Dementia

Introduction

1. Patients may present with rapidly progressing dementia or with previously undiagnosed insidious progression of cognitive impairment
2. Diagnosis
   a. helps with prognostication/family planning
   b. ideally identifies some reversible cause

Questions to Ask

1. What is the timeline of the cognitive decline?
   a. rapid progression makes Alzheimer's type dementia less likely
   b. if sudden change, may be due to recent illness, medication change
   c. use acronym VITAMINS for differential diagnosis of rapidly progressive dementia
      i. vascular
      ii. iatrogenic
      iii. toxic-metabolic
      iv. autoimmune
      v. infectious
      vi. neurodegenerative/neoplastic
      vii. systemic processes

2. Have there been any recent changes in medications?
3. Is there a family history of early dementia/dementing process?
4. Screening for nutritional deficiencies
   a. Any changes in diet over time?
   b. Any history of alcohol abuse?
5. Are there parkinsonian features?
   a. clues to Lewy body dementia and other parkinsonian diseases
6. Is there urinary incontinence?
   a. normal pressure hydrocephalus triad of dementia, shuffling/magnetic gait and incontinence rare but important to recognize
7. Is there a history of depression?
   a. depression may present as "pseudodementia"
   b. consider more formal screen/psychiatry evaluation
8. Has there been a stepwise progression over time?
   a. may indicate vascular dementia from multiple strokes

Exam Findings

1. mental status exam
   a. Mini Mental Status Exam (MMSE) is good for screening and for comparison over time in patients with Alzheimer's disease
2. Careful neurological examination looking for any evidence of focality/asymmetry
   a. Evaluate for other chronic neurological diseases (e.g., Parkinson's)
3. Thorough general physical examination for evidence of systemic disease/malignancy

Diagnostic Tests

1. Labs
   a. CBC
   b. CMP—electrolytes and hepatic function screening
   c. TSH
   d. B12 levels
   e. cortisol
   f. RPR or VDRL to screen for syphilis
   g. HIV
2. Imaging
   a. CT brain
      i. less sensitive than MRI
   b. MRI brain
      i. preferable study for dementia
      ii. more sensitive for subtle abnormality
      iii. patterns typical of specific types of dementia may be apparent
3. Lumbar puncture
   a. if prolonged time course of limited utility
   b. excludes inflammatory disorders (e.g. sarcoid, CNS vasculitis, CNS infection)
   c. may help diagnose Creutzfeldt Jakob disease (send for 14–3–3 protein although very non-specific)
      i. diagnosis largely clinical however
4. EEG
   a. limited utility but may show specific patterns helpful in diagnosis

Treatment Options

1. Correct underlying cause if identified
2. Medications

a. Typically neurologist-directed
b. As appropriate if any of the above conditions diagnosed

When to Consider Consulting a Neurologist

1. For most newly diagnosed dementia, as an inpatient or in follow-up

Care Transitions

1. Assure appropriate placement
2. Close neurologist/primary care follow-up as indicated

Proposed Quality Metrics

1. Fall rates
2. Formal care pathways in place to decrease development of delirium

Coma and Brain Death

Questions to Ask

1. Is the patient comatose, stuporous, or encephalopathic?
   a. coma
      i. lack of alertness and awareness with eyes closed
      ii. broad range of etiologies
      iii. can result from anesthesia, drugs, or structural, infectious, inflammatory etiologies
      iv. typically these patients have a Glasgow Coma Scale (GCS) of 8 or less (Table 18.1)
   b. stupor
      i. depressed level of consciousness
      ii. typically patients will follow commands only after stimulation by loud voice or noxious stimuli
   c. Encephalopathy
      i. synonymous with delirium
      ii. alteration of attention
      iii. typically patients will follow basic verbal commands
      iv. may be hypoactive or hyperactive
      v. may have features of tremor, asterixis, and/or myoclonus if associated with organ dysfunction (e.g., liver, renal, thyroid failure)
2. What neuroanatomic components create consciousness?
   a. consciousness requires components of alertness and awareness

TABLE 18.1 The Glasgow Coma Scale (Teasdale and Jennett 1974)

Eye-opening response
- 4 Spontaneous
- 3 To speech
- 2 To painful stimulus
- 1 None

Best motor response in upper limbs
- 6 Obeys commands
- 5 Localizes
- 4 Withdraws (normal flexion)
- 3 Flexes abnormally (spastic flexion)
- 2 Extends
- 1 None

Verbal response
- 5 Oriented
- 4 Confused
- 3 Inappropriate words
- 2 Incomprehensive sounds
- 1 None

The Glasgow coma score can be used in patients of all ages and is reproducible between different observers (Teasdale et al. 1978). The *best verbal* component of the scale needs to be adjusted to take into account the age of children, particularly under five years (Reilly et al. 1988). The best post-resuscitation Glasgow coma score is used to classify severity of head injury. The severity of craniocerebral injury is classified as:
- mild, Glasgow coma score from 15 to 13;
- moderate from 12 to 9; and
- severe, 8 or less.
Reprinted with permission of Donaghy M, Brain's Diseases of the Nervous System: Cerebrovascular Diseases. Oxford University Press.

b. awareness- multiregional brain integration of multiple brain regions that lead to awareness of environment
c. alertness
   i. phenotype of eye opening
   ii. primarily a function of the reticular activating system (RAS) in the brainstem with projections to bilateral thalami and bilateral hemispheres

3. What are important categories of coma and altered states of consciousness?
   a. coma, stupor, and encephalopathy can be transient or permanent depending on the underlying etiology
   b. vegetative patients may be alert but are not aware
   c. persistent vegetative state (PVS) requires
      i. at least 4 weeks of a vegetative state
      ii. no medication or metabolic confounders
      iii. typically occurs after severe traumatic brain injury (TBI) or anoxia (diffuse brain injury)
      iv. described as "wakeful unconsciousness" since they appear alert but are not aware (cortical integration).
   d. minimally conscious state (MCS)
      i. typically occurs in patients similar to PVS
      ii. is distinguished by the presence of definitive awareness of self or environmental, which is NOT present in PVS
      iii. may follow commands (albeit intermittentky)
   e. locked-in state (LIS)
      i. may appear that patient is not following commands in extremities
      ii. have normal consciousness
      iii. can typically blink, or make vertical (up or down gaze) eye movements to command
      iv. typically caused by bilateral ventral pontine lesions (vertebrobasilar occlusion or pontine hemorrhage)
      v. important to screen for this on examination in patients supposedly in coma
4. What is brain death?
   a. irreversible and total loss of all brain and brainstem function
5. How do you prognosticate after cardiac arrest?
   a. exercise great caution prior to 48–72 hours except in cases of brain death
   b. predictors of poor neurologic outcome (PVS or death at 3 months or 1 year)

     i. absent pupillary reflexes on day 1 and 3 of cardiac arrest

    ii. absent GCS motor response on day 1 (in patients not made hypothermic) and day 3 after hypothermia and sedation/paralysis stopped

      1. GCS motor scale < 3 (flexor posturing or worse) on day 3 is particularly suggestive of possible poor outcome, but not 100% specific

      2. caution is advised about this sign in those who received hypothermia due to possible lingering sedation and/or neuromuscular paralysis. Therefore, more time may be required in hypothermia cases

   iii. somatosensory evoked potentials (SSEP)

      1. neurophysiologic test in which the median nerve or tibial nerve is stimulated and the cortical N20 response is assessed over the cortex

      2. SSEP N20 potentials when absent have been shown (in technically adequate study) to be highly specific to poor outcome (100%) especially prior to hypothermia

   iv. EEG

      1. nonspecific unless shows suppression-burst pattern or "myoclonus status epilepticus"

      2. This has a high 99–100% specificity for poor outcome at least in the prehypothermia era

    v. serum neuron-specific enolase (NSE)> 33ng/ml measured 24–72hrs post arrest

      1. associated with poor outcome (specificity 85%)

      2. lack of widespread availability

      3. lab turnaround times may preclude its use

      4. unlear impact of hypothermia on results

6. Determination of brain death criteria:

  a. neurological intracranial catastrophe (either primary such as massive intracranial bleeding, TBI, or stroke, or secondary after cardiac arrest and global brain hypoxia)

  b. no confounding factors to affect the neurological examination

   i. sedating medications
   ii. paralytics
   iii. hypothermia (< 36C core temp)
   iv. profound electrolyte disturbance (e.g. serum sodium < 125, or > 155)
c. not following any verbal commands and no evidence of locked-in state
d. absent brainstem reflexes
   i. pupillary
   ii. corneal
   iii. oculocephalics (doll's eyes)
   iv. oculovestibular (cold-water calorics)
   v. cough/gag
   vi. not breathing above ventilator rate
e. apnea test (apneic oxygenation)
   i. last confirmatory step in brain death testing
   ii. patient is preoxygenated with 100% FiO_2 for 15minutes,
   iii. patient has no contraindications or expectations to desaturate coming off ventilator (large A-a gradient, flail chest, pulmonary edema, with high PEEP, FiO_2 requirements)
      1. if no contraindications and after preoxygenation, patient is taken off ventilator to exclude ventilator self-cycling from hyperdynamic flow triggering
   iv. patient has SBP >95mmHg (pressors allowed)
   v. 6–8L/min FiO_2 delivered at carina via cannula. Note higher cannula flow rates (8L/min) may reduce $PaCO_2$ rise during apnea test
   vi. Baseline ABG targets normocapnea ($PaCO_2$ – 35–40mmHg), ventilator adjustment may need to be made
   vii. confirmatory findings are increase in $PaCO_2$ 20mmHg above 40mmHg baseline, or to absolute above 60mmHg

viii. If patient too unstable from pulmonary standpoint to undergo apnea test, ancillary confirmatory brain death confirmatory testing may include

1. EEG recorded at 2uV sensitivity showing complete flatline (suppression)
2. TCD assuming good temporal windows, showing no intracranial flow, or if flow only "short spikes" or reverberating flow
3. SPECT scan, showing "hollow skull": no intracranial uptake of brain parenchyma
4. cerebral angiogram shows no intracranial flow above the carotid (intracranial) terminus

Other Exam Findings

1. General approach to the comatose patient
   a. ABCs—stabilize the patient
      i. GCS 8 or less, consider intubation for airway protection
   b. neck immobilization if history of trauma
2. Neurological examination
   a. Glasgow Coma Scale (GCS)
      i. a simple scale that helps define these roughly
      ii. does not supplant the full neurological examination
   b. mental status
      i. ask the patient to look up or down, blink eyes to screen for locked-in state
   c. cranial nerve examination helps localize damage to the brainstem or above
      i. localizing helps determine site of the lesion and potential prognosis
      ii. the pons typically controls horizontal gaze centers

iii. the midbrain cranial nerve III and vertical gaze integration

d. flexor posturing (decorticate) typically indicates damage or injury above the red nucleus

e. extensor (decerebrate) posturing typically indicates damage below the midbrain (red nucleus)

Diagnostic Tests

1. Labs
   a. CBC for occult infection
   b. CMP/hepatic panel
   c. always check a glucose
   d. TSH screening
   e. toxicology screening—for drugs of abuse, tricyclic overdose if applicable, and other drugs based on the history
   f. anti-epileptic drug levels—in patients with epilepsy
2. Imaging
   a. consider noncontrast CT of the brain to exclude intracranial structural abnormalities such as ICH, SAH, SDH, or tumor
   b. consider MRI
      i. if CT is inconclusive and if no other clear cause identified
      ii. especially if there are brainstem findings on neurological examination to suggest posterior circulation ischemia, posturing
3. EEG—if the initial tests above are negative to evaluate for nonconvulsive seizure
4. Lumbar pucture
   a. if no other clear etiology
   b. especially with fever, leukocytosis
   c. in the immunocompromised

Treatment Options

1. Treatment is specific to the underlying etiology
   a. For CNS stroke and intracranial hemorrhage, see ICH chapter, ICP chapter
   b. For drug overdose, consider reversal agents
      i. many of these are non-specific
      ii. narcotic overdose, narcan administration
      iii. benzodiazepine overdose, flumazenil administration
      iv. coma with opthalmoplegia in nutritionally-deficit patient, consider thiamine administration
   c. for meningitis, perform LP and start empiric antibiotics
   d. most comatose patients are admitted to an ICU environment and if intubated, supported with mechanical ventilation until improvement, or if permanent neurologically injured, prognostication and discussion with family or proxy about health care/life support wishes are clarified

When to Consider Consulting a Neurologist

1. Unclear coma etiology
2. EEG testing or SSEP
3. Neurologic prognostication
4. Abnormal neurological findings

Care Transitions

1. Comatose patients typically stay in the ICU environment unless they improve and can be extubated
2. Stuporous and encephalopathic patients benefit from multicomponent interventions for delrium; see delirium chapter for detail

Other Considerations

1. Aspiration prevention
   a. head of bed elevation 30–45 degrees
   b. in intubated patients
      i. daily sedation vacation if possible
      ii. oral cleansing measures by nursing and/or respiratory staff
2. DVT prevention
   a. sequential/progressive compression devices
   b. subcutaneous heparin or heparinoids for DVT prevention if no neurological (ICH) contraindications
3. Alcohol withdrawal seizures—typically do not need anti-epileptic medications. CIWA or similar benzodiazepines may be indicated and thiamine replacement

Proposed Quality Metrics

1. Comprehensive coma evaluation and examination as above are performed in a timely manner and documented
2. In patients who are febrile, with meningitic signs, time to LP and empiric antibiotic and steroid administration is considered
3. In septic comatose patients, early antibiotic administration
4. In cardiac arrest patients who are successfully resuscitated, initiation of therapeutic hypothermia (32–34C x 12–24hrs) within 6hrs of arrest if stable to improve neurologic outcomes and overall survival
5. Thiamine administration in alcoholic and nutritional deprived individuals before dextrose administration to prevent/exacerbate Wernicke's encephalopathy/Korsakoff syndrome

6. Prevention of falls in the hospital
7. Foley removal as soon as possible to prevent catheter-associated UTI
8. Removal of central lines as soon as possible
9. Early screening for delirium and multicomponent intervention

19

Approach to and Management of the Patient with Weakness

Questions to Ask

1. Is the onset of weakness acute, subacute or chronic (or acute on chronic)?
   a. acute weakness suggests an acquired process such as
      i. acute neuromuscular AIDP (acute inflammatory demyelinating polyradiculopathy or Guillain-Barré syndrome or GBS)
      ii. vascular (stroke or spinal cord injury)
      iii. inflammatory (vasculitis, especially if painful)
      iv. toxic (heavy metal poisoning)
   b. subacute to chronic suggests a progressive disease such as
      i. neuropathy
      ii. myopathy (e.g., statin/HMG CoA)
      iii. myasthenia gravis (painless)
      iv. inflammatory myositis (especially if painful)
      v. infiltrative (amyloidosis)
      vi. anterior horn cell disease such amyotrophic lateral sclerosis (ALS)
2. Is there a history of weakness before hospitalization?
   a. history of a neuromuscular diagnosis such as
      i. myotonic dystrophy (or muscular dystrophy in the family)
      ii. myasthenia gravis

   iii. Guillain-Barré

   iv. CIDP (chronic inflammatory demyelinating poly-neuropathy)

   v. peripheral neuropathy?

  b. Is there a history of porphyria (acute exacerbations can cause acute multifocal mononeuropathy often with abdominal pain)?

3. What are the two major levels in the nervous system that cause weakness?

 a. a critical question as this guides the evaluation

 b. central nervous system (CNS)

  i. typically contralateral face and arm weakness if lesion is within the hemispheres or basal ganglia

  ii. crossed if at the brainstem (face and limb weakness are opposite sides)

  iii. upper motor neuron (UMN) findings usually occur from CNS lesions:

   1. weakness (corticospinal tract pattern)

   2. hyperreflexia

   3. upgoing toe (Babinski) or Hoffman's sign (hand middle finger nail flick stimulation causes hyperactive thumb flexion reflex)

 c. peripheral nervous system (PNS)

  i. typically reduced reflexes in a root distribution or diffuse (neuropathy)

  ii. lower motor neuron (LMN) findings

   1. weakness (radicular, muscle pattern, neuromuscular junction)

   2. hyporeflexia

   3. hypotonia

   4. fasciculations

4. What is the pattern of weakness?

 a. bilateral lower extremity weakness

      i. if chronic, most commonly due to distal symmetrical neuropathy as from diabetes

  b. generalized weakness

      i. raises concern for Guillain-Barré syndrome (often ascending)

     ii. generalized myasthenia (if no sensory symptoms and ocular, bulbar involvement)

    iii. botulism

    iv. toxic ingestions

      1. heavy metals

      2. thallium toxicity

      3. arsenic

      4. lead

      5. buckthorn berry ingestion

     v. tick paralysis

    vi. diphtheria toxin in those with preceding upper respiratory symptoms

   vii. CMV polyneuropathy in immunocompromised hosts

  viii. AIDS/HIV

      1. polyneuropathy

      2. CMV

      3. EBV

5. Was pain a feature of weakness?

  a. if so, consider vasculitis or myositis

6. Is the patient taking any medications that cause weakness?

  a. corticosteroids

  b. statins

  c. d-penicillamine

  d. HIV medications

      i. zidovudine

     ii. stavudine

    iii. lamivudine

  e. amiodarone

  f. aminoglycosides

g. quinolones

h. quinidine

i. verapamil

j. phenytoin

k. interferon-alpha

l. sulfamethoxazole and trimethoprim

m. quetiapine

n. paralytics

    i. vecuronium

    ii. pancuronium

    iii. cisatricurium

7. Does the patient have a history of diplopia?

    a. can be a subtle sign of preexisting weakness of many causes

    b. commonly described in myasthenia gravis

8. Has the patient been critically ill?

    a. critical illness myopathy

        i. seen in failure to wean from ventilator

        ii. diffuse weakness

    b. critical illness polyneuropathy

        i. includes sensory deficits as well

    c. may need both EMG/nerve conduction studies and muscle biopsy to diagnose

    d. associated especially with sepsis and paralytic use

9. Has the patient been on steroids?

    a. may present acutely but typically insidious onset of myopathy

    b. more proximal than distal weakness

10. Was the patient exposed to any environmental or infectious causes?

    a. West Nile virus infection (mosquito vector) causes asymmetric flaccid weakness due to anterior horn cell-like degeneration, sometimes with encephalitis

b. snake bite envenomation
   i. antivenom can be considered but the type of snake must be described or ideally captured (alive or dead)
   ii. coral snake ("red & yellow kill a fellow") contiguous red and yellow markings
      a. myokymia (intermittent irregular twitching of eyelid or other muscle without weakness) and fasciculations
      b. myokymia/fasciculations of the chest may be heralding sign before sudden respiratory failure
   2. Rattle snakes
      a. antivenin can be given for concern for severe envenomation syndrome but rest is supportive; hydration, short-term hospitalization
c. Marine toxins (ingested):
   i. ciguatoxin (fish contaminated with dinoflagellates "red tide")
      1. GI symptoms
      2. muscle aches and weakness
      3. sensory symptoms often predominate
   ii. saxitoxin (shellfish)
      1. numbness
      2. diffuse severe weakness which can progress to respiratory failure and death if not supported by mechanical ventilation
   iii. tetrodotoxin (puffer fish)
      1. GI symptoms
      2. paresthesias
      3. diffuse muscle weakness, which may present as rapid ascending paralysis occurs by 24 hours which starts in the extremities, then bulbar muscles and finally respiratory muscles
      4. Reflexes are preserved early in the course of paralysis
      5. Because of CNS toxicity, coma and seizures are reported, and even loss of all brain stem reflexes

    d. buckthorn berry ingestion—Guillain-Barré-like syndrome

    e. heavy metals: arsenic, gold, thallium

        i. can mimic Guillain-Barré-like weakness

        ii. diagnose with 24hr urine heavy metal screening

    f. pesticides: organophoshates—cholinergic symptoms

Exam Findings

1. Clinical examination

    a. cranial nerve examination

        i. ptosis, fatiguability, lid lag, for myasthenia gravis

        ii. tongue strength as assessment for bulbar function and swallow capability

    b. neck flexion strength as a surrogate for C2 muscular/diaphragmatic strength/respiratory function

    c. motor examination (MRC motor scales)

        i. MRC 0—no movement to gravity

        ii. MRC 1—trace muscle movement (on visual inspection or palpation)

        iii. MRC 2—movement with gravity eliminated

        iv. MRC 3—movement is stronger than gravity

        v. MRC 4 (can be +/-) movement stronger than gravity and has some resistance against examiner

        vi. MRC 5—normal strength to resistance

    d. upper motor neuron (UMN) findings

        i. weakness

        ii. spasticity (may take hours or days to develop) after stroke or other acute CNS lesion

        iii. hyperreflexia

        iv. corticospinal tract weakness—typically contralateral weakness in face (lower) and extremities in stroke. Ipsilateral to lesion below level of the medullary decussation (e.g., cervical spine)

        1. select spinal cord patterns
           a. Brown-Séquard contralateral pain loss, ipsilateral motor loss
           b. anterior cord syndrome, preserved vibration and proprioception, but flaccid plegia of the lower extremities if lower than C8 spinal cord level, with associated pain and temperature loss; typically from vascular spinal cord injury

  e. lower motor neuron (LMN) findings
     i. weakness
     ii. hypotonia (reduced tone)
     iii. reflexes usually reduced
     iv. dermatomal or radicular (spinal root) weakness or sensory loss
     v. bilateral pattern
        1. neuropathy
        2. deconditioning
        3. myasthenia—weakness, especially when fatiguable (better in A.M. or after rest, worse after exertion or later in day); reflexes are typically preserved
        4. Guillain-Barré
           a. sensory loss and weakness common
           b. diffuse hyporeflexia or areflexia is a clinical hallmark
           c. lumbar puncture typically shows normal WBC and elevated protein (cytoalbuminemic dissociation).
     vi. fasciculations

  f. sensory examination
     i. Light touch in face and extremities as a screen
     ii. "Stocking glove" pattern is consistent with length-dependent neuropathies such as diabetes and other polyneuropathies
     iii. dermatomal sensory examination especially in those with spinal cord history to localize sensory levels (Figure 19.1)

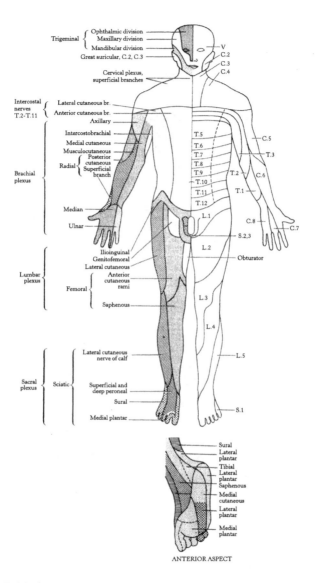

FIGURE 19.1

Dermatome Map. Reprinted with permission of Watson M, Oxford Handbook of Palliative Care. Oxford University Press.

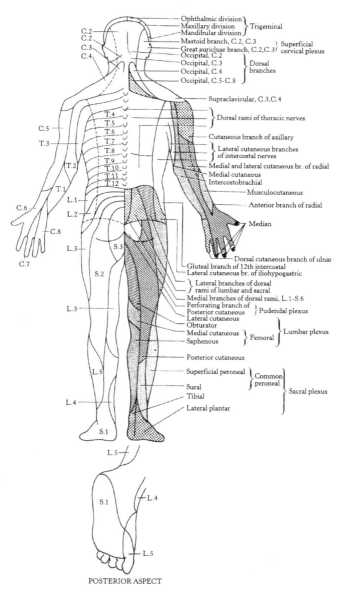

FIGURE 19.1 (Continued)

Diagnostic Tests

1. Imaging
   a. if weakness is unilateral or crossed (face on one side and body on the other)
      i. suggests CNS involvement
      ii. CT of the brain is suggested (without contrast to exclude stroke)
      iii. followed by MRI
   b. if weakness is bilateral, then clinical findings should classify as UMN or LMN
      i. UMN patterns of weakness suggest CNS (neuroimaging of brain or spinal cord) or may (rarely) suggest anterior horn cell disease (ALS) which has both LMN and UMN findings
   c. MRI preferred for the spinal cord to evaluate for compression or ischemia
   d. if a trauma patient, often CT spine imaging is performed first to exclude gross fractures and misalignment
2. Labs—overall yield likely low
   a. electrolyte abnormality
      i. sodium and calcium usually low yield, unless sodium overcorrection in central pontine myelinloysis
      ii. magnesium toxicity can cause weakness through the neuromuscular junction
      iii. phosphorous deficiency can precipitate rhabdomyolysis
   b. serum glucose (always assure that this has been done)
   c. serum CK
      i. rhabdomyolysis
      ii. myositis
      iii. compartment syndrome
   d. toxicology screening
   e. if inflammatory disorder suspected

        i. CRP

       ii. sedimentation rate

     iii. possible anti Jo1 antibodies (myositis such as polymyositis/dermatomyositis)

     iv. CK

      v. ANA (antinuclear antibody) panel

  f. if myasthenia gravis suspected

       i. AChR- acetylcholine receptor antibodies

      ii. if asymmetric or with an unusual history

         1. ganglioside antibodies (GM1 ganglioside levels)

  g. GQ1B antibodies for Miller Fisher syndrome (ataxia, ophthalmoplegia, and areflexia)

  h. anti-epileptic drug levels—in patients with epilepsy

  i. lumbar puncture

       i. consider in immunocompromised

      ii. infection of uncertain cause

     iii. suspected GBS

     iv. persistently abnormal mental status

3. EMG

  a. useful in LMN processes

  b. in critical illness polyneuropathy or myopathy, it is more confirmatory of the clinical diagnosis or sometimes prognostic if the weakness is severe (axonal neuropathy pattern vs. demyelinating)

  c. may not be abnormal acutely

4. Muscle/nerve biopsy—if there is a specific question such as myositis, congenital myopathy, or vasculitis

Treatment Options

1. Specific to each disorder—for example, diabetic neuropathy best treated with ideal glucose control

2. GBS (also known as acute inflammatory demyelinating polyradiculopathy, AIDP)
   a. in nonambulatory cases, IVIG 0.4g/kg/day IV x 5 days (caution in IgA deficient patients as anaphylaxis reported) of Guillain-Barré
   b. Plasma exchange (PLEX): for severe GBS cases involving respiratory function or deteriorating rapidly, PLEX x 5 days is often used due to its faster onset of action than IVIG; requires Quentin size central venous catheter and 5 days treatment
   c. Advantages and disadvantages of each approach are debated
3. Myasthenia gravis
   a. First line (non-crisis): Corticosteroids carefully up titrating to 1mg/kg/day dose and bridging to a steroid sparing agent like azathioprine (Imuran) or mycophenolate mofetil
   b. Myasthenic crisis: (involves respiratory function)
      i. IVIG and plasma exchange are also immunomodulatory therapies
      ii. similar to GBS, rapid respiratory involvement, PLEX works faster in removal of antibodies, and treatment is 5 days
4. Polymyositis/dermatomyositis
   a. hydration
   b. corticosteroids

When to Consider Consulting a Neurologist

1. Unclear cause of weakness
2. Many of these disorders, especially when in crisis
3. EMG request
4. Specific medications dosing or regimen

Care Transitions

1. Assure education about safety issues at discharge
2. Review driving/reporting issues specific to your state
3. Transitioning to follow-up care of neurological diagnosis in hospital (e.g., myasthenia gravis)
4. Home health therapies as appropriate

Other Considerations

1. For patients being placed on chronic corticosteroids consider
   a. osteoporotic prevention with calcium and vitamin D supplementation, fosamax weekly or equivalent
   b. PCP (Pneumocystis carinii) prophylaxis
   c. gastric ulcer prevention with famotidine or ranitidine.
2. Physical therapy and occupational therapy to prevent weakness and help with balance, gait, and strengthening
3. DVT prevention especially in those with limited mobility

Proposed Quality Metrics

1. DVT prevention
2. Physical, occupational therapy consultation
3. Speech language pathology consultation
4. AIDP- time to receive IVIG once diagnosed and not ambulatory
5. Statin medication review and those associated with weakness

Parkinson's Disease/Parkinsonism

Questions to Ask

1. Does the patient have an established dosing regimen for their Parkinson's disease medications?
   a. patients will often have spent years in adjusting medications
   b. very sensitive to changes in medication doses, schedules and formulations
   c. schedules and doses may be difficult
      i. to enter into EMR systems
      ii. for pharmacy to supply
      iii. ideally, systems set up ahead of time to facilitate
      iv. with newer drugs, may need families to bring in medications
2. Is there a history of delirium?
   a. these patients are at high risk of delirium
   b. many Parkinson's medications increase this risk
   c. subtle or clinically inapparent dementia lowers threshold for delirium
3. Is there an increased risk of falls?
   a. typically in the highest risk category
   b. take appropriate precautions
4. Does the patient have a known diagnosis of Parkinson's disease?
   a. Parkinsonism
      i. similar clinical features but secondary to drugs or other cause
      ii. may be difficult to differentiate from Parkinson's disease

      iii. many potential drugs implicated (Table 20.1)
         1. phenothiazines
         2. butyrophenones (haloperidol)
         3. benzamides (metoclopramide)
         4. valproic acid
         5. verapamil
         6. lithium
      iv. other medical conditions
         1. CNS infections
         2. head trauma
         3. other neurodegenerative diseases

Exam Findings

1. Bradykinesia—motor slowing
2. Flat affect/masked facies
3. Rest/pill rolling tremor
4. Postural instability
5. Soft voice
6. Cogwheel type rigidity

Diagnostic Tests

1. Imaging—unnecessary for diagnosis
2. Lumbar puncture—consider if CNS infection a concern
3. Labs—none specific

Treatment Options

1. Parkinson's disease
   a. NPO patients
      i. levodopa/carbidopa intestinal gel

TABLE 20.1 Drugs associated with Parkinsonism

Dopamine receptor blocking drugs

'Older' anti-psychotics
- Chlorpromazine
- Haloperidol
- Flupentixol
- Sulpiride
- Pimozide
- Trifluoperazine

'Atypical' anti-psychotics
- Quetiapine
- Clozapine
- Risperidone
- Olanzapine
- Amisulpiride
- Sertindole
- Zotepine

Others
- Metoclopramide
- Prochlorperazine

Dopamine depleting drugs
- Tetrabenazine

Other drugs
- Cinnarizine
- Fluphenazine
- Lithium
- Amiodarone
- Sodium valproate
- Diltiazem

      ii. apomorphine

      iii. dopamine patch

    b. routinely institute aspiration precautions

    c. low threshold for swallow evaluation

    d. delirium and fall minimizing protocols

  2. Other causes of Parkinsonism

    a. stop offending medication(s)

    b. dopamine agonists and other Parkinson's disease medications may be helpful

When to Consider Consulting a Neurologist

1. Low threshold to consult especially if diagnosis uncertain
2. Perioperative medication management
3. Behavioral difficulty
4. Prolonged NPO periods for Parkinson's disease patients

Care Transitions

1. Assure optimal medication reconciliation both on admission and discharge

Other Considerations

Proposed Quality Metrics

1. Adherence to established medication schedules
2. Avoidance of falls/fall rates
3. Avoidance of delirium
4. Lengths of stay impacted by falls/delirium
5. Documentation of discussion of ramifications of feeding tube placement

Dystonic Reactions

Questions to Ask

1. What is a dystonic reaction?
   a. spasmodic/sustained uncomfortable contractions
   b. reversible extrapyramidal symptoms
   c. may be caused by medications, toxins, trauma, encephalitis, metabolic disorders or stroke
2. Is this a dystonic reaction?
   a. typically acute onset
   b. abnormal posturing and movements
   c. mostly head/neck
   d. commonly painful
3. Has the patient started on any new medications? (Figure 21.1)
   a. calcium channel blockers
   b. neuroleptics
   c. toxin exposures (cocaine)
   d. tricyclic antidepressants
   e. general anesthetics
   f. ranitidine
   g. compazine

Exam Findings

1. Contractions, typically painful

- Dopamine receptor blocking drugs
- Amine depletors (e.g. tetrabenazine)
- Antidepressants: serotonin-reuptake inhibitors, monoamine oxidase inhibitors
- Calcium antagonists
- Benzodiazepines
- General anaesthetic agents
- Anti-convulsants (carbamazepine, phenytoin)
- Triptans
- Ranitidine
- Cocaine
- Ecstasy

FIGURE 21.1

Commonly reported causes of acute dystonic reactions

Diagnostic Tests

1. Clinical exam is diagnostic

Treatment Options

1. Anticholinergics—first line
   a. benztropine
   b. diphenhydramine
2. Benzodiazepines
3. Parkinson's medications may be helpful
   a. trihexyphenidyl
   b. dopamine agonists
4. Stop offending medication(s)
5. Monitor patient for 24 hours

When to Consider Consulting a Neurologist

1. Low threshold to consult especially if diagnosis uncertain

Care Transitions

1. Assure follow up if medication changes have been made (e.g., psychiatric medications)

Neoplastic Disorders

Introduction

1. Brain tumors
   a. metastatic tumors to the brain are more common than primary brain tumors: metastases are more often multiple in number
      i. common from lung, breast, and colon cancer especially
      ii. certain tumors are prone to hemorrhagic metastases: melanoma, thyroid, renal cell, choriocarcinoma
   b. Primary brain tumors
      i. malignant: glial cell-derived are the most common
         1. low grade glioma (WHO Grade II)
         2. anaplastic astrocytoma (WHO Grade III)
         3. glioblastoma multiforme (WHO Grade IV)
      ii. primary CNS lymphoma
         1. in patients with immunosuppression (esp. HIV)
         2. in immune competent patients
      iii. benign: meningioma is the most common benign primary brain tumor and is found incidentally on many imaging studies
2. Carcinomatous meningitis
   a. much less common than brain metastases and associated with an extremely poor prognosis
3. Malignant spinal cord compression

a. in patients with widely metastatic cancer, the incidence approaches 5%
b. arises from extension of metastatic disease from the bony spine most typically

Questions to Ask

1. Is there a history of progressive neurologic deficits over weeks to months?
2. Headaches are common with intracranial neoplasm and may have features of increased intracerebral pressure (ICP) including worsening with lying flat and awakening the patient from sleep
3. Is there a history of systemic malignancy personally and/or in the family?
4. Especially when considering CNS lymphoma, a history of HIV and its risk factors should be elicited
5. Bladder function should be assessed in patients with suspected spinal cord compression including nighttime frequency and incontinence

Exam Findings

1. Evidence of focal findings localizing to the central nervous system
2. Papilledema suggesting increased intracranial pressure
3. With suspected carcinomatous meningitis, often multiple cranial nerves or spinal roots will be affected
   a. Neck stiffness is a relatively uncommon finding but should be assessed
4. When spinal cord compression is suspected, looking for signs of bowel and bladder dysfunction is important

a. tenderness over the midline spine may suggest vertebral body involvement

b. assessing for a "spinal cord level" below which sensation is diminished on the trunk will allow for determination of the cord level that is involved

Diagnostic Tests

1. Imaging
   a. MRI with contrast is typically the test of choice for identifying tumors of the brain and spinal cord
      i. high-grade glial neoplasms often demonstrate ring enhancement, although other processes such as infection (bacterial abscess, toxoplasmosis) and subacute hemorrhage can also have this appearance
      ii. meningiomas typically arise from the dura and homogeneously enhance
      iii. imaging of the spinal cord allows for direct visualization of tumor pressing against the spine in suspected cord compression
   b. systemic imaging with CT of the chest/abdomen/pelvis, perhaps in conjunction with PET scan, may be helpful in patients to screen for systemic malignancy if metastases or other CNS complications of systemic cancer are suspected
2. Labs
   a. HIV testing for patients with suspected lymphoma
   b. if systemic lymphoma is suspected: SPEP, UPEP, LDH
   c. rarely will systemic tumor markers be useful
3. Biopsy
   a. tissue diagnosis typically the key test for brain tumor diagnosis
   b. in cases of suspected metastases, a systemic site is usually more accessible to biopsy than one in the CNS

4. Lumbar Puncture
   a. should only be attempted if patient is not at risk for herniation
   b. CNS lymphoma
      i. typically demonstrates lymphocytic pleocytosis, often with high protein
      ii. EBV PCR can be useful to make the diagnosis of CNS lymphoma in HIV+ patients but not in immunecompetent patients
      iii. CSF cytology and flow cytometry can make the diagnosis of lymphoma but are insensitive tests, even when using high volumes of CSF
         1. Repeat testing (x3) is a reasonable step to improve sensitivity
   c. Carcinomatous meningitis
      i. Typically demonstrates lymphocytic pleocytosis, often with high protein and low glucose
      ii. CSF cytology should be sent on a high volume of fluid that is delivered promptly to the lab (fresh specimen)

Treatment Options

1. Initial management
   a. if the patient demonstrates evidence of elevated ICP
      i. consider osmotic agents such as mannitol
      ii. consider corticosteroid administration with dexamethasone
         1. note that corticosteroids can affect the diagnostic yield in CNS lymphoma and therefore should be avoided if at all possible
   b. for malignant spinal cord compression
      i. begin corticosteroids immediately with dexamethasone
   c. Seizures should be treated with anticonvulsants

2. Brain tumor
   a. treatment dependent on the type and grade of the tumor
   b. brain metastases
      i. surgery for solitary lesion
      ii. radiation is the mainstay of therapy
   c. high-grade glial neoplasms: surgery followed by radiation and chemotherapy (temozolomide most commonly)
   d. CNS lymphoma: typically treated with radiation and chemotherapy, NOT surgical resection
   e. meningioma: conservatively managed unless causing symptoms or growing, in which case surgical resection is the mainstay of therapy
3. Carcinomatous meningitis
   a. focal radiation to sites of disease
   b. consideration of chemotherapy, often delivered intrathecally
4. Malignant spinal cord compression
   a. emergent surgery or emergent radiation therapy are the mainstays of treatment to avoid progressive disability, especially when the symptoms are relatively new in onset (<72 hours)

When to Consider Consulting a Neurologist

1. In the workup of an unknown brain lesion(s)
2. Suspected spinal cord compression
3. Seizures

Care Transitions

1. Patients often require referral to a practitioner with a neurooncology background for further treatment

   a. Radiation oncology and/or neurosurgery may also be involved depending on the tumor type and treatment plan

2. Advise against driving for those who have experienced seizures

Proposed Quality Metrics

1. Patients with malignant spinal cord compression should be urgently treated with surgery or radiation therapy if deficits are new or rapidly progressive
2. Biopsy of CNS mass should occur in cases of suspected malignancy without systemic involvement and otherwise negative workup

Paraneoplastic Neurologic Disorders

Introduction

An increasingly recognized group of disorders affecting mainly the central nervous system that are malignancy-related but not caused by direct involvement of tumor

1. Caused by antibodies directed against cell surface antigens (e.g., NMDA receptor encephalitis)
   a. tend to have a better prognosis when treated
2. Caused by antibodies directed against intraneuronal antigens (e.g., anti-Hu encephalitis)
3. Some peripheral nervous system disorders including neuropathy, myasthenia gravis and Lambert-Eaton myasthenic syndrome may also occur

Questions to Ask

1. Is there a known systemic malignancy?

Exam Findings

1. Patients can present with a variety of symptoms but central nervous system paraneoplastic syndromes should be considered especially in the setting of seizures, psychiatric illness, or unexplained meningitis

Diagnostic Tests

1. Imaging
   a. MRI may be normal but may also demonstrate hyperintensities in the temporal lobes ("limbic encephalitis") or other areas of the brain
   b. PET/CT to look for systemic malignancy
      i. of note, tumors causing these neurologic syndromes are often small and in early stages
      ii. small cell lung CA the most common malignancy but these syndromes have been described with a variety of other malignancies including breast, ovarian, testicular, and other adenocarcinomas
   c. pelvic ultrasound or pelvic MRI
      i. useful in NMDA-receptor encephalitis in young women to screen for ovarian teratoma
      ii. useful in anti-Yo cerebellar disease in young women to screen for ovarian carcinoma
2. Biopsy
   a. tissue diagnosis of systemic malignancy can be helpful
3. Lumbar puncture
   a. almost always (>90%) abnormal with either (1) elevated lymphocytes, (2) oligoclonal bands unique to CSF, or (3) elevated IG index; the latter two tests must be sent in conjunction with serum studies
4. Labs
   a. serum (or less commonly CSF) paraneoplastic panels can be helpful for definitive diagnosis
      i. if specific syndrome or malignancy is suggested, more directed testing can ensue
5. EEG if seizures suspected

Treatment Options

1. Initial management
   a. anticonvulsants should be administered if seizures have occurred
2. Treatment/removal of underlying tumor is the most effective therapy
3. Immunomodulation
   a. steroids
   b. plasmapheresis or intravenous immunoglobulin
   c. B-cell depleting chemotherapies

When to Consider Consulting a Neurologist

1. In any suspected paraneoplastic neurologic syndrome

Care Transitions

1. Patients will require referral to neurology
   a. in many cases, recovery from the neurologic syndrome may lag behind treatment of the malignancy by several weeks or months and therefore close neurologic follow-up required
2. Advise against driving for those who have experienced seizures

Proposed Quality Metrics

1. Consider paraneoplastic disorders in cases of unexplained neurologic dysfunction or encephalitis
2. Systemic screen for malignancy should be undertaken with CT or PET/CT

24

Visual Disturbances

Questions to Ask

1. Is the vision loss monocular or binocular?
   a. monocular vision loss is typically caused by diseases affecting the eye, globe, retina, and optic nerve; unilateral vision loss is typically not due to brain visual pathway disease
   b. binocular vision loss typically involves the brain, chiasm, or the bilateral visual pathways in temporal, parietal or occipital lobes (Figure 24.1)
2. Was the vision loss or disturbance: painful or painless?
   a. painless vision loss is common in occipital or retinal ischemia from embolism
   b. painful vision loss is suggested of "arteritic" (vasculitic) optic nerve ischemia such as giant cell arteritis or optic neuritis
3. Was the visual disturbance transient or persistent?
   a. amaurosis fugax is the term for transient monocular vision disturbance or loss from ipsilateral carotid disease
   b. persistent vision loss should be classified as monocular or binocular and visual field deficit should be mapped
4. Was the onset acute or gradual?
   a. acute monocular disorders
      i. typically suggest optic nerve ischemia
      ii. Ophthalmology consultation is very helpful in confirming optic nerve ischemia or inflammation

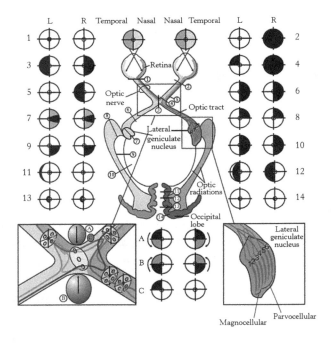

FIGURE 24.1

Visual Pathways

    iii. arteritic ischemic optic neuropathy (AION): synonymous with giant cell (temporal arteritis) and other vasculitic disease that cause ischemia to optic nerve head

    iv. non-arteritic ischemic optic neuropathy (NAION)

        1. non-vasculitic causes of anterior ischemic optic neuropathy such as atherosclerotic disease and carotid disease

        2. Hollenhorst plaques/emboli may be seen

        3. evaluation as with stroke

            a. atherosclerotic disease (vascular carotid +/- intracranial arteries)

            b. echocardiography if concern for cardiac embolism

        4. treatment typically with risk factor modification (blood pressure, glycemic, and lipid control) and antithrombotics for secondary prevention

    v. optic neuritis

        1. autoimmune inflammation of the optic nerve typically in young, female patients

        2. may be precursor to multiple sclerosis (or overlap disease)

        3. typically sudden painful vision loss in young patient

        4. treatment with corticosteroids

    vi. orbit issues

        1. vitreal bleeding

        2. retinal detachment

b. acute binocular events suggest brain ischemia affecting one of the visual pathways (see Figure 24.1)

    i. homonymous hemianopia

        1. common in occipital lobe lesions which affects half of the side of the vision

        2. lesions which affect the optic radiations to the occipital lobe (Figure 24.1, lesion number 6)

    ii. bitemporal hemianopia suggests chiasmal disease (Figure 24.1, lesion number 3)

    iii. homonymous quadrantanopia suggest posterior visual pathways and

        1. either temporal lobe (Meyer's loop, "pie in the sky" pattern (Figure 24.1, lesion number 8)

        2. or medial parietooccpital lobe, "pie on the floor" (Figure 24.1, lesion number 9)

c. gradual onset disorders suggest more indolent processes

    i. if monocular

        1. orbit disease

          a. cataract

          b. glaucoma

          c. retinal disease

       d. diabetic retinopathy

       e. macular degeneration

    2. inflammatory disease

       a. sarcoidosis

    3. compression

       a. tumor (Figure 24.1, lesion numbers 1 and 2)

  ii. if binocular

    1. most commonly in chiasmal bitemporal hemianopic pattern

    2. lesions of the pituitary region (sella, parasellar region) that cause chiasmal blindness—mnemonic SATCHMO

       a. S: sarcoidosis, sellar tumor (pituitary adenoma, prolactinoma)

       b. A: aneurysm (internal carotid or anterior communicating artery)

       c. T: teratoma, tuberculosis ("tuberculoma")

       d. C: craniopharyngioma, cyst (Rathke's cleft cyst, clival chordoma

       e. H: hypothalamic lesion (glioma, hamartoma of tuber cinereum), and histiocytosis X

       f. M: meningioma, metastasis

       g. O: optic nerve glioma (neurofibromatosis, type I or II)

       h. (Figure 24.1, lesion number 3, and inset of chiasmal lesions with differential chiasmal compression A, B, and C)

Exam Findings

1. Visual field examination

  a. patient stares at stationary object in distance or at examiner's nose and object presented in the periphery to detect vision loss

    b. this can be done binocularly or monocularly (closing or covering one eye), the latter of which allows for more precise localization

2. Visual acuity if the complaint is vision loss
    a. perform using the patient's glasses if available
3. Reading, writing testing for alexia and agraphia
    a. functions that connect visual cortex association cortex to language areas
4. Fundoscopic examination to examine for optic neuropathy
    a. can cause a pallor or edema of the optic disc
    b. Hollenhorst plaques
    c. branch retinal artery occlusion
    d. retinal or vitreal hemorrhage
    e. papilledema
5. The eye should be examined with a slit lamp for trauma or foreign body if there is suggestive history
6. Standard neurological exam to screen for other deficits to help localize the injury
7. Temporal arteries may be palpated for beading and tenderness (giant cell arteritis), although these signs are insensitive for the disease

Diagnostic Tests

1. Imaging
    a. CT brain is suggested if the visual field deficit localizes to the brain (hemianopia)- stroke, hemorrhage, tumor, etc
    b. if CT is inconclusive, and pattern still suggests brain pathology, MRI should be obtained
    c. if orbital pain is present or exophthalmos seen, CT or MRI of the orbits may disclose mass, enhancement (optic neuritis), or extraocular muscle pathology (e.g. Grave's disease)

2. Labs
   a. sedimentation rate in those suspected of giant cell arteritis
   b. complete blood count if anemia is suspected
   c. infectious serologies: Bartonella henselae (cat scratch) if history suggestive and neuroretinitis present
3. Tonopen
   a. Measurement of eye pressure in patients with suspected or known glaucoma to exclude acute angle closure and elevation in intraocular pressure (IOP)

Treatment Options

1. Monocular vision loss with elevated sedimentation rate
   a. consultation with an ophthalmologist, vascular surgeon, or neurosurgeon for temporal artery biopsy (possible giant cell arteritis)
   b. start the patient on corticosteroids (1gram Solu Medrol daily or high dose oral steroids (1mg/kg) x 3 days) immediately unless there is a contraindication. This can be followed by 60mg prednisone po daily
2. For HSV eye infection, acyclovir or valacyclovir should be urgently initiated

When to Consider Consulting a Neurologist or Ophthalmologist

1. Unexplained vision loss: neurologist if binocular, ophthalmologist if monocular; both require emergent attention
2. Stroke or other brain lesion: neurologist

Care Transitions

1. Educate about safety issues, especially driving in visually impaired patients by discharge
2. Review driving/reporting regulations specific to your state
3. Neurologist or ophthalmologist follow-up as needed
4. Home safety evaluation

Other Considerations

1. Fall precautions are important in visually impaired
2. Physical/occupational therapy evaluation for a gait aid and gait stability

Proposed Quality Metrics

1. Obtaining biopsy and starting steroids immediately for suspected giant cell arteritis
2. Documentation of education of fall and driving precautions as well as safety issues prior to discharge
3. Appropriateness of neuroimaging

Vertigo and "Dizziness"

Questions to Ask

1. Did the patient experience vertigo or "dizziness?"
   a. Patients with vertigo often feel as if they were moving
      i. most often described as a spinning sensation
   b. Patients with other causes of dizziness may also describe
      i. "feeling like I was going to pass out" may indicate a presyncopal episode
      ii. "I feel dizzy when walking" might indicate disequilibrium from a variety of causes
      iii. "I felt lightheaded" may make a clinician suspect hyperventilation or other causes of nonspecific dizziness
2. Describe the episode
   a. When asking patients to describe the episode, one should use open-ended questions to allow the patient to fully describe the episode
      i. each answer should then be clarified in an effort to obtain as much specificity regarding the symptoms as possible
   b. What were you doing at the time?
   c. Did you feel as if you were going to "pass out?"
3. How long have you had the symptoms?
   a. vertigo is usually self-limited
   b. chronic dizziness, lasting longer than several weeks, is usually due to other causes of dizziness (e.g., psychiatric, hyperventilation, impaired balance)

4. Was there anything that prompted the symptoms?
   a. postural changes
   b. walking
   c. emotional or other triggers
5. Does changing positions trigger the feeling?
   a. vertigo is always made worse with head movement
      i. patients with vertigo will often lie very still in an effort to prevent the symptoms from occurring
6. Have you had any changes with your hearing?
   a. may imply a peripheral cause of the vertigo
7. Have you had any nausea or vomiting?
   a. can be a worrisome finding, indicating a central vestibular lesion
   b. one should ask the patient if they are also having symptoms of slurred speech, incoordination, and double vision

Exam Findings

1. Vital signs
   a. orthostatic hypotension may point one in the direction of a presyncopal episode, either due to intravascular depletion, diurectic use or anti-hypertensives (i.e., beta blockers)
   b. tachycardia, bradycardia or arrhythmia may indicate cardiac etiology
2. Gait instability
   a. if the patient has a unilateral peripheral abnormality, they will usually lean or fall toward the affected side
3. Evidence for a central lesion
   a. eye movements
      i. patients complaining of dizziness with nystagmus most likely have vertigo

      ii. gaze-evoked horizontal nystagmus (with or without a torsional component) which limits after a few beats may indicate a peripheral cause of vertigo

      iii. vertical nystagmus should point one toward a central cause

      iv. a patient with a central cause of their syncope will *not* have their nystagmus suppressed by visual fixation

      v. nystagmus from central vertigo typically does not fatigue as quickly as peripheral

   b. other cranial nerve abnormalities

      i. evaluate each cranial nerve carefully

      ii. hearing—abnormality may point to a peripheral cause

   c. coordination helpful, especially looking for evidence of a cerebellar/posterior circulation process

Diagnostic Tests

1. Dix-Hallpike maneuver (Figure 25.1)
   a. performing this maneuver:
      i. sit the patient at the edge of the bed
      ii. rapidly move the patient to the lying position, supporting their head
         1. the head should be turned 45 degrees to one side and tilted downward 45 degrees
   b. the development of nystagmus and vertigo with the maneuver establishes benign positional vertigo as the cause of the patient's symptoms *if* the symptoms match what the patient has described

2. Orthostatics
   a. a decrease in systolic blood pressure > 20mmHg and diastolic blood pressure > 10mmHg following standing. The heart rate should increase with standing

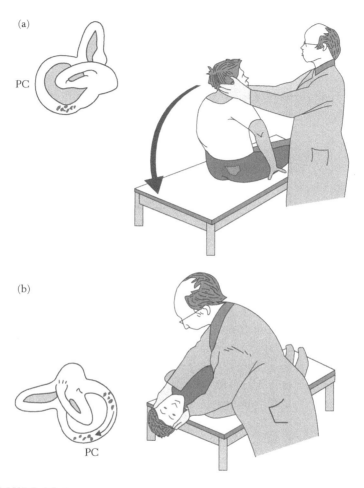

FIGURE 25.1

Dix-Hallpike Maneuver

3. Evaluation of hearing
   a. Weber test
      i. a vibrating tuning fork is placed in the middle of the patient's forehead
      ii. normal patients will hear the sound equally in both ears
      iii. patients with conductive hearing loss will hear the tuning fork louder in the affected ear
      iv. patients with sensorineural hearing loss hear the tuning fork better in the normal ear
   b. Rinne test
      i. a vibrating tuning fork is placed on the mastoid process just behind each ear
      ii. when the sound is no longer heard, the tuning fork is moved just outside the ear itself
      iii. in a normal ear (positive Rinne test), the air conduction is greater than the bone conduction
         1. bone conduction greater than air conduction indicates a conductive hearing loss
   c. identification of sensorineural hearing loss is suggestive of a peripheral cause of the patient's symptoms
4. MRI should be performed if there is concern for a central lesion causing vertigo

Treatment Options

1. Treatment will be based upon the underlying etiology
2. Medication classes:
   a. antihistamines
      i. these are the most commonly used medications in patients with vertigo
      ii. meclizine is the most common and has been demonstrated in some older studies to have some benefit
      iii. the medications are usually well tolerated

  iv. anticholinergic side effects can be a problem, especially in elderly patients
 b. antiemetics
  i. these medications are more sedating than the antihistamines
  ii. they are good for patients with vertigo and significant nausea/emesis
 c. benzodiazepines
  i. sedation is a problem with these medications
  ii. they are most often used in patients with vertigo who cannot take antihistamines
3. Canalith repositioning maneuver
 a. the Dix-Hallpike test establishes which side is affected
 b. the Epley maneuver is a method of repositioning the canalith which is causing symptoms (Figure 25.2)
  i. turn the patient's head 45 degrees to the involved side
  ii. hold the patient's head with two hands and recline the patient to a supine position, head hanging over the edge of the bed
  iii. keep the patient's head in this position until nystagmus or symptoms improve (roughly 30 seconds)
  iv. turn the patient's head 90 degrees away from the affected ear and allow vertigo to resolve (roughly 30 seconds)
  v. help the patient roll up onto their shoulder and keep the head at the sam orientation (face 45 degrees to the floor) and wait another 30 seconds
  vi. maintain the same head position and assist the patient in sitting up, wait at least 30 seconds before moving
  vii. may be repeated if needed
4. Vestibular exercises
 a. patients should be referred to therapists specifically trained in vestibular rehabilitation
 b. vestibular rehabilitation can improve patient symptoms and postural confidence

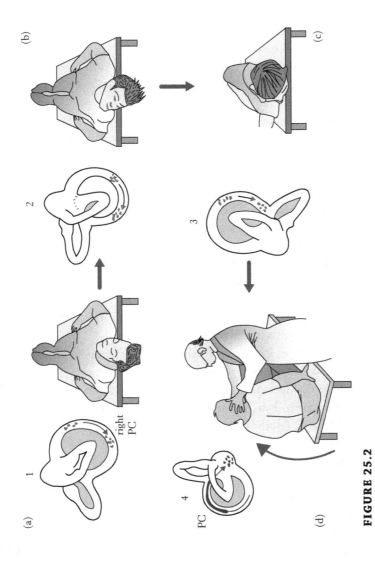

FIGURE 25.2

Canalith Repositioning (Epley) Maneuver

When to Consider Consulting a Neurologist

1. Focal neurologic deficit
2. Concern for central lesion
3. Uncertain diagnosis

Care Transitions

1. Patients with peripheral vestibular dysfunction should be referred for vestibular rehabilitation as an outpatient
2. Careful fall precautions, especially in the elderly
3. If the patient is admitted and there is a concern for central cause, admit with frequent neurological checks

Proposed Quality Metrics

1. Performance and documentation of key parts of the physical examination
2. Utilization of diagnostic imaging
3. Were fall precautions used especially for elderly patients?
4. Referral to vestibular rehabilitation

Other Spinal Cord Processes

Questions to Ask

1. What are clues to spinal cord processes?
   a. back pain (but spinal cord etiology for back pain is very uncommon)
   b. sensory level—examine along cervical/thoracic/lumbar/sacral spine for differences in sensation
   c. bowel/bladder dysfunction
   d. history of underlying tumor or other risk factor
2. When is it appropriate to consult a neurosurgeon/spine surgeon?
   a. early consultation in cases of impending or evident neurologic compromise is critical
3. What is transverse myelitis?
   a. an (often demyelinating—see demyelinating processes chapter 9) inflammation of the spinal cord
   b. pathogenesis/etiology unclear, but may follow viral or bacterial infection or in those with underlying autoimmune disease
   c. symptoms depend on area involved, can be across an entire (transverse) level of the cord
   d. may be an acute or subacute process associated with pain and paresthesias

Exam Findings

1. A careful neurological exam is essential
2. A general physical exam with attention to evidence of trauma or malignancy
3. Motor exam
   a. may be able to define level of involvement
   b. important to test gait if able to do so
   c. rectal tone a potentially important clue
   d. may note muscle wasting due to lower motor neuron damage
4. Sensory exam
   a. testing along both sides of the back from sacrum to neck
   b. findings may be subtle
5. Reflexes
   a. asymmetry a clue
   b. may help establish level

Diagnostic Tests

1. Imaging
   a. MRI is most sensitive (Figure 26.1)
   b. CT an alternative, intravenous contrast needed
   c. plain X rays may be helpful for bony disease but relatively insensitive
      i. fractures
      ii. metastatic disease
2. Lumbar puncture
   a. low yield and potential to introduce infection/tumor into intradural space
3. Labs
   a. blood
      i. CBC to evaluate white count/differential

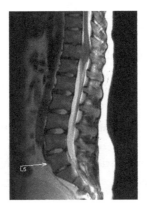

FIGURE 26.1

MRI showing cord impingement from a tumor at T11

      ii. ESR typically elevated
      iii. C reactive protein usually elevated
      iv. transverse myelitis
          1. autoimmune workup
          2. B12 level
          3. infectious workup (HIV, RPR, etc.)

Treatment Options

1. Admit patients with cervical cord disease or risk for progressive disease to a closely monitored unit
2. Spinal cord injury due to blunt trauma
   a. much debate over steroid utility in spinal cord injury
      i. typically 30mg/kg bolus administered within 8 hours
      ii. followed by 5.4 mg/kg/hr for 23 hours
   b. surgical intervention as appropriate

3. Tumor compression
   a. dexamethasone 10 mg IV, then 4 mg q6 hours
   b. radiation/surgery depending on type of tumor
4. Transverse myelitis
   a. little rigorous data but tailored to cause
   b. for autoimmune disease: typically methylprednisolone 1gm/day for 3–5 days

When to Consider Consulting a Neurologist

1. Low threshold to consult especially if diagnosis uncertain
2. Concern for neurological abnormalities on examination
3. Cases of transverse myelitis

Care Transitions

1. Follow-up with rehabilitation services as appropriate
2. Follow-up with neurology in transverse myelitis for possible demyelinating disease (eg., multiple sclerosis)

Other Considerations

1. Physical and occupational therapy
2. Physiatry consultation

Proposed Quality Metrics

1. Documentation of full neurological exam
2. Timeliness of imaging
3. Initiation of appropriate spine precautions
4. Timeliness of appropriate consultations

Glossary

abulia—diminished drive or initiative

anterior horn cell—alpha motor neuron cell bodies that control axial muscles

apraxia—inability to perform a task despite having the physical ability to do so

aphasia—impairment of ability to speak and/or understand despite the motor ability to do so

areflexia—absent reflexes

ataxia—unsteady, discoordinated motor movement

chiasmal—relating to the optic chiasm—the crossing of the optic nerves

cogwheeling—increased muscle tone characterized by a ratcheting sensation to the examiner

coma—lack of alertness and awareness with eyes closed

corpus callosum—white matter tracts that connect the two cerebral hemispheres

corticospinal tract—descending motor nerves

craniopharyngioma—a cystic suprasellar neoplasm

dysarthria—slurring of the speech, different from aphasia

encephalopathy—alteration of attention, like delirium

fasciculations—involuntary palpable or visible muscle contractions

graphesthesia—able to recognize what is written or traced on the skin

Hollenhorst plaques—cholesterol/atheromatous emboli that lodge in the retinal arterial system, may be visible on ophthalmoscopic evaluation

leukoariosis—areas of the brain with a characteristic appearance on neuroimaging, related to small vessel ischemia

lower motor neuron—neurons that innervate skeletal muscles

myositis—muscle inflammation

myotonic dystrophy—common muscular dystrophy affecting adults, related to a trinucleotide repeat, characterized by prolonged muscle relaxation

ophthalmoplegia—ocular muscle paralysis

papilledema—optic disc edema, may be a sign of increased intracranial pressure

polyradiculopathy—a process affecting multiple nerve roots

proprioception—the ability to discern the relative positions of parts of the body

stereognosis—ability to recognize an object by touch

stupor—depressed level of consciousness

supratentorial—above the tentorium cerebelli

transcranial doppler (TCD)—ultrasound that is able to evaluate flow in portions of the intracranial arteries

uncus—the parahippocampal gyrus which is vulnerable in the setting of herniation

upper motor neuron—neurons that help form the corticospinal tract, connecting to the lower motor neuron

vegetative state—lack of awareness of self and environment, sleep-wake cycles are present

Appendix

The ABCD2 Tool for Transient Ischaemic Attack

Criteria	Point system
A Age	1
B Blood pressure ≥140/90 mmHg	1 point for hypertension at the acute evaluation
C Clinical features	2 points for unilateral weakness, 1 for speech disturbance without weakness
D Symptom Duration	1 point for 10–59 min, 2 points for ≥60 min
D Diabetes	1 point

Important Myotomes

Muscle*	Roots	Nerve	Action
Trapezius	C3, 4	Spinal accessory	Shrug shoulder
Rhomboids	C4, 5	Dorsal scapular	Brace shoulders back
Supraspinatus	C5, 6	Suprascapular	Abduct shoulder 15°
Deltoid	C5, 6	Axillary	Abduct shoulder 15–90°
Infraspinatus of arm	C5, 6	Suprascapular	External rotation
Biceps	C5, 6	Musculocutaneous	Flex forearm
Triceps	C6, 7	Radial	Extend forearm
Extensor carpi	C5, 6	Radial	Extend wrist
Finger extensors	C7, 8	Posterior interosseous	Extend fingers
FDP I and II	C8, T1	Median	Flex DIPJ
FDP III and IV	C8, T1	Ulnar	Flex DIPJ
FDS	C8, T1	Median	Flex PIPJ
APB	C8, T1	Median	Abduct thumb
OP	C8, T1	Median	Thumb to 5th finger
ADM	C8, T1	Ulnar	Abduct 5th finger
1ST DIO	C8, T1	Ulnar	Abduct index finger
Iliopsoas	L1, 2	Femoral	Flex hip
Hip adductors	L2, 3	Obturator	Adduct hip
Hip extensors	L5, S1	Inferior gluteal	Extend hip
Quadriceps	L2, 3	Femoral	Extend knee
Hamstrings	L5, S1	Sciatic	Flex knee
Tibialis anterior	L5, S1	Deep peroneal	Dorsiflex foot
Gastrocnemius	S1, 2	Tibial	Plantarflex foot
Tibialis posterior	L4, 5	Tibial	Invert foot
EHL	L5, S1	Deep peroneal	Dorsiflex hallux
Peroneus longus	L5, S1	Superficial peroneal	Evert foot

*Muscles in bold font are essential in a basic neurological examination.

Dermatomes

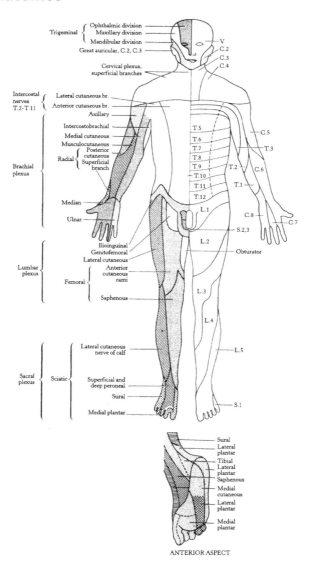

ANTERIOR ASPECT

Dermatomes (Continued)

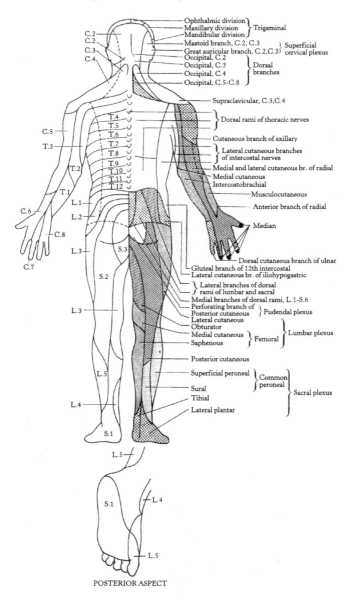

Ophthalmic division ⎫
Maxillary division ⎬ Trigeminal
Mandibular division ⎭
Mastoid branch, C.2, C.3 ⎫ Superficial
Great auricular branch, C.2,C.3 ⎭ cervical plexus
Occipital, C.2 ⎫
Occipital, C.3 ⎬ Dorsal
Occipital, C.4 ⎭ branches
Occipital, C.5-C.8

Supraclavicular, C.3, C.4

Dorsal rami of thoracic nerves

Cutaneous branch of axillary

Lateral cutaneous branches
of intercostal nerves

Medial and lateral cutaneous br. of radial
Medial cutaneous
Intercostobrachial
Musculocutaneous
Anterior branch of radial
Median

Dorsal cutaneous branch of ulnar
Gluteal branch of 12th intercostal
Lateral cutaneous br. of iliohypogastric
Lateral branches of dorsal
rami of lumbar and sacral
Medial branches of dorsal rami, L.1-S.6
Perforating branch of ⎫
Posterior cutaneous ⎬ Pudendal plexus
Lateral cutaneous ⎭
Obturator ⎫
Medial cutaneous ⎬ Femoral ⎫ Lumbar plexus
Saphenous ⎭ ⎭

Posterior cutaneous

Superficial peroneal ⎫ Common
⎬ peroneal ⎫ Sacral plexus
Sural ⎭
Tibial
Lateral plantar

POSTERIOR ASPECT

The Glasgow Coma Scale (Teasdale and Jennett 1974)

Eye-opening response
- 4 Spontaneous
- 3 To speech
- 2 To painful stimulus
- 1 None

Best motor response in upper limbs
- 6 Obeys commands
- 5 Localizes
- 4 Withdraws (normal flexion)
- 3 Flexes abnormally (spastic flexion)
- 2 Extends
- 1 None

Verbal response
- 5 Oriented
- 4 Confused
- 3 Inappropriate words
- 2 Incomprehensive sounds
- 1 None

The Glasgow coma score can be used in patients of all ages and is reproducible between different observers (Teasdale et al. 1978). The *best verbal* component of the scale needs to be adjusted to take into account the age of children, particularly under five years (Reilly et al. 1988). The best post-resuscitation Glasgow coma score is used to classify severity of head injury. The severity of craniocerebral injury is classified as:
- mild, Glasgow coma score from 15 to 13;
- moderate from 12 to 9; and
- severe, 8 or less.

Index